UY
(Gib)

RUGBY MEDICINE

Proceedings of an International Conference

EDITED BY

TERENCE GIBSON
MD, FRCP
Consultant Physician, Guy's Hospital,
St Thomas' Street, London

AND

JOHN DAVIES
MRCS, LRCP, DPhys Med
Consultant in Physical Medicine
and Rehabilitation,
Harley Street Sports Clinic,
London

WITH THE COMPLIMENTS OF

LEDERLE LABORATORIES

BLACKWELL SPECIAL PROJECTS
OXFORD

© 1991 by
Blackwell Scientific Publications
(Blackwell Special Projects)
Editorial Offices:
Osney Mead, Oxford OX2 0EL

First published 1991

Set, printed and bound
at The Alden Press, Oxford

DISTRIBUTORS

Marston Book Services Ltd
PO Box 87
Oxford OX2 0DT
(*Orders*: Tel: 0865 791155
Fax: 0865 791927
Telex: 837515)

British Library
Cataloguing in Publication Data

Rugby medicine.
I. Gibson, Terence
II. Davies, John
617.1027

ISBN 0-632-03338-X

FRONT COVER. Dr Ben Gilfeather attends to Ieuan Evans who has dislocated a shoulder.
Lions tour of Australia 1989. Photo courtesy Colorspot.

Contents

Contents

Contents

[vii]

List of Contributors

B.W.D.BADLEY MD, FRCP, FRCPC, *Professor of Medicine, Dalhousie University, Halifax, Nova Scotia, Canada; former Chairman, Refereeing and Laws Committee, Canadian Rugby Union, Canada (Correspondence: Victoria General Hospital, 1278 Tower Road, Halifax, Nova Scotia, Canada B3H 2Y9)*

H.C.BURRY FRCP, FRACP, *Professor and Director of Rehabilitation Medicine, The Amalgamated and Essenden Hospitals, Grafton Street, Parkville, c/o Post Office, The Royal Melbourne Hospital, Victoria 3050, Australia*

J.CHASE MD, FACS, *Medical Adviser and Injury Consultant, 425 28th Street, Oakland, California 94710, USA*

P.CUNNINGHAM MB, ChB, *Fellow, New Zealand Federation of Sports Medicine, 28 Tiri Road, Milford, Auckland 9, New Zealand*

J.E.DAVIES MRCS, LRCP, DPhys Med, *Honorary Physician, Welsh Rugby Union, and Medical Director, Harley Street Sports Clinic, 110 Harley Street, London W1N 1AF, UK*

P.ENGLAND FRCS, *Member of the Rugby Football Union Injuries Working Party; Consultant Orthopaedic Surgeon, Hammersmith and North Middlesex Hospitals, London, UK; and 73 Harley Street, London W1N 1DE, UK*

T.GIBSON MD, FRCP, *Consultant Physician, Guy's Hospital, London SE1 9RT, UK*

B.GILFEATHER, MB, ChB, DRCOG, *Medical Officer to the Rugby Football Union, 279 Farnham Road, Slough, Berkshire SL2 1HA, UK*

S.GRAY MS, PhD, *Associate Professor, Department of Recreation and Leisure Studies, California State University, Sacramento, 6000 J Street, Sacramento, California 95819–6110, USA*

E.GRAYSON MA(Oxon), *Barrister and Consultant to the Sports Council and the Central Council for Physical Education, 4 Paper Buildings, Temple, London EC4Y 7EX, UK*

C.HAMMOND MB, ChB, DSports Med, *Sports Physician, Sports Medical Centre, PO Box HM1425, Hamilton HMFX, Bermuda*

List of Contributors

E.P.HUGO *Chairman, South African Rugby Medical Association, and Consultant Orthopaedic Surgeon, PO Box 11431, Brooklyn 0011, Republic of South Africa*

I.KONO MD, PhD, *Associate Professor, Division of Sports Medicine, Institute of Health and Sports Sciences, University of Tsukuba, 1 Chome 1-1, Tennodai, Tsukuba, Ibaraki 305, Japan*

G.R.McLATCHIE FRCS, *Consultant Surgeon, The General Hospital, Hartlepool TS24 9AH, UK*

M.MOLLOY MB, FRCP, *Honorary Medical Officer, Irish Rugby Football Union, and Consultant Rheumatologist and Lecturer in Medicine, University College, Cork Regional Hospital, Wilton, Cork, Eire*

M.O'BRIEN FRCPI, *Professor, Department of Anatomy, Trinity College, Dublin 2, Eire*

S.D.W.PAYNE FRCS (Ed and Eng), *The Medical Protection Society, London W1, and Department of General Surgery, Central Middlesex Hospital, London NW10, UK*

J.PENE MD, *Physician to the French Rugby Union, 118/119 Cours D'Alsace et Lorraine, Bordeaux 33000, France*

J.C.M.SHARP MB, ChB, FFPHM, MRCP(Glas.), *Consultant Epidemiologist, Communicable Diseases (Scotland) Unit, Ruchill Hospital, Glasgow G20 9NB, Scotland*

J.P.R.WILLIAMS MBE, FRCSEd, *Consultant Orthopaedic Surgeon, Princess of Wales Hospital, Coity Road, Bridgend, Mid-Glamorganshire CF3 11RQ, Wales*

Introduction

RUGBY is a sport which inherently poses some risk of physical injury. Robust encounters, controlled collision and football skill are the features which characterise an activity which is unashamedly masculine. This element of sporting hazard is not unique to rugby and it is an aspect which enhances its challenge to participants. The attitudes of society to physical confrontation and danger in sport change with time and it behoves all relevant authorities to maintain an awareness of what is popularly and legally acceptable. In this context rugby has evolved. As players have become fitter, faster and stronger the risks of serious injury arising from deliberate or accidental collision and other body contact have increased. To this has also been added an increased competitiveness which may have enhanced the vigour with which games are played. Modifications of the rugby laws and changes in playing techniques and tactics may also influence adversely or otherwise the potential for injury. These are the reasons why it is essential for doctors to be involved in the development of rugby; to monitor the patterns of injury with time, to alert the governing authorities to unacceptable hazards and practices, to ensure that players' medical problems receive prompt diagnosis and treatment and to educate administrators, coaches and players in the avoidance and management of injury.

The game has been historically associated with the medical profession through the medical schools. Guy's Hospital RFC in London is the oldest rugby club in the world, being formed in 1843. Since those days, members of the medical profession have won honours at international level and continue to do so, in many countries.

In recent years, there has been increasing awareness and recognition of sports medicine as a specialty. Higher postgraduate education and diploma programmes are common world-wide. In the UK, the Royal College of Physicians and Surgeons of Glasgow, and the Royal College of Physicians and Surgeons of Edinburgh have created a Board of Sport and Exercise Medicine together with an examination for a postgraduate Diploma of Sports Medicine. It has taken many years of intense lobbying for the establishment of postgraduate training and examination in health matters appertaining to a sporting population.

Sports medicine is fragmented world-wide, and with an ever increasing list of sport and leisure pursuits together with seemingly endless paramedical involvement in the specialty, attaining meaningful information within the medical profession is extremely difficult. To work at one sport at a time, each with its peculiar and particular problem areas would be far more rewarding and satisfying.

It was with this in mind that the International Conference on Rugby Medicine was organized. In the last few years, many countries have organized their own rugby medicine associations and the Japanese Kento Medical Society is especially prolific in membership and scientific output. Argentina, Italy, France and South Africa have similar associations.

Doctors and other interested parties from 13 different rugby playing countries assembled in Bermuda between 11th and 15th November 1990. It was intended that the proceedings and recommendations should be published and circulated prior to the Rugby World Cup competition in 1991. The impetus and organisation of the meeting were entirely the results of the efforts of Dr John E. Davies.

Communication and cross-fertilisation of ideas can only help to eradicate potential problem areas. Perhaps we should be thinking along the lines of an international association of rugby doctors, such as an international college of rugby medicine, working with and reporting to the world governing body, the International Rugby Board. Existing rugby medicine associations could have representation, and centralisation and collation of rugby medicine data and clinical information world-wide would be of invaluable assistance to the game's administrators.

Rugby medicine has arrived, and it is only fitting that through its historical association with the game, the medical profession is answering many of the questions regarding the authenticity and acceptance of sports medicine, by exercising preventative medicine in the team sport it helped to create.

There was much informal discussion which went unrecorded at the conference but the principal sessions together with their associated discussions have been collated and edited to form this publication. We hope that the contents enjoy a wide readership amongst doctors, officials, players and commentators. The editors wish to thank Julian Grover and Blackwell Scientific Publications for their forbearance during the publication of the book and wish to acknowledge their debt to the Lederle Pharmaceutical Company whose sponsorship has made it possible. The Bermuda Conference was supported by BUPA, Pfizer Pharmaceutical Co., Medisport

Introduction

International, Prisma Ltd, The Sportcare Foundation and the United States Rugby Football Foundation. To all of these we express our sincere thanks.

J.E.DAVIES, T.GIBSON
London, July 1991

PART 1
THE EPIDEMIOLOGY
OF INJURY

1: The Value of
Rugby Injury Surveys

PATRICK ENGLAND

In the last century, the sport of kings was likened to the image of war without its guilt. The allusion could be equally well applied to rugby. The game of football originated in the Dark Ages and has been banned on a number of occasions in the UK by various kings because of the difficulties and injuries that occurred. Unfortunately no statistics on this survive.

In 1984, the Rugby Football Union formed an injuries working party and gave terms of reference which were as follows: (a) to be responsible for advising the Rugby Football Union on any matter which may prevent or reduce the incidence of injury within the game; (b) to start some simple forms and protocol; and (c) to begin a feasibility study which took place in the first season. There are many rugby-playing clubs, school (units), some of whom may have more than three teams. It was therefore decided to confine the study to the first three XVs of each unit included and to take note that many schools only play one term of football.

In order to conform with the Data Protection Act, a unique code number was allocated to each club, the record of which was kept by the injuries co-ordinator. Each player, as he was injured, was also given a unique number, a record of which was kept at the club.

We looked at the age range, where the injuries occurred in the game, how the management of the injury was disposed of and the effect on play. We also looked at the occupation of the players.

The instructions for entry were simple. Proformata were sent once a month to a central individual who was responsible for collating them and passing them on to be programmed onto the computer. We invited 100 clubs to participate.

Not only are players tired but frustration creeps in towards the end of the game, particularly in league matches. The pilot study revealed a phenomenal number of deliberate injuries in the beginning of the game. We attributed this to players getting to know each other and determining their friends. At the beginning of the second half there seemed to be a resurgence which faded. These accounted for roughly 10% of injuries. However, in later studies, the deliberate injuries were sustained throughout the game and we question whether the introduction of league competitiveness contributed to this.

The scrum was associated with a low incidence of injury and the majority occurred in open play, tackling or being tackled. This was consistent over a number of years of study. Technique in tackling and falling is important.

In one year, two very serious neck injuries leading to paralysis occurred when nobody was near the player at all. On the first occasion, the full-back was running back to collect the ball coming over his head, he stumbled and fell forward with head in flexion. In the second, a player was simply running forward to rejoin the game when he stumbled, fell forward and broke his neck.

Results from the 1988–89 and 1989–90 seasons suggest that the scrum is almost the safest place to be, other than the line-out, where the risks seemed least. There was only one fractured skull reported in the whole of the series. The head and neck injuries were largely cuts and contusions. There have only been one or two eye injuries. The highest range of incidence was in those players aged between 19 and 30. The incidence of shoulder injuries varies from 9 to 13%. During the season, particularly in 1985–86, the frequency of all injuries was highest at the beginning of the season. The condition of the pitch seemed to have no influence. A small number were advised off the game medically. More people gave up voluntarily after an injury.

Neck injuries represent the only situation in which a denominator population can be applied and is the only injury which is really, statistically meaningful. Our data are insufficient, but the accumulated aggregates show that the pattern in each sample was roughly the same, except in neck injuries where there was a definite trend downwards. The denominator population is the same in each year for neck injuries, because it is mandatory for these to be reported to the Rugby Football Union. In the 1985–86 season there were 29 injuries reported and one which we found unreported. There was only one serious injury from eight due to collapsing scrums. Two injuries resulted in tetraplegia. There have been 2 years in which none was reported. In the season 1989–90 there was only one permanent injury. There were 30 neck injuries, four were serious and only one resulted in permanent tetraplegia, the others being temporary. One needed a spinal fusion, two had temporary braces, and two have resumed rugby.

There was a low percentage of injury in the front row. The back row (the flankers) seemed the most vulnerable. In the early phase of the studies it was the wing who was most prone but with time the centres seemed more likely to suffer.

[4]

There were 403 hospital treatments reported out of some 996 injuries in 1989–90 but there were only 156 attendances. Of these, 24% were admitted and there was a low incidence of serious injury or operation. The total number of days in hospital was 225.

We estimated that over 5 of 6 years, a very serious injury occurred in about 4: that is one injury per 146.5 hours. It seems that the bigger the sample, the less the chance of being injured.

The cumulative injuries over three or four seasons showed a similar pattern.

An important message from the statistics is that fitness is all. We really must be fit in order to play the game. One must not play the game to get fit. Technique is also important and one has to be taught and to practise the techniques, otherwise injuries will occur. The laws are crucial and the referee is important.

2: Rugby Injuries in Canada

BERNARD W.D.BADLEY

ALTHOUGH injuries are inevitable in a sport such as rugby football, several recent reports have expressed concern over the continued occurrence of serious injuries [1–5] despite the introduction of law changes designed to reduce the incidence of such injuries. The current study was initiated by the Refereeing and Laws Committee of the Canadian Rugby Union in order to determine the type and frequency of injuries in Canadian rugby, to indicate the phases of play in which injuries most commonly occur, and to consider whether additional law changes might be expected to reduce the incidence of injuries.

For the purposes of this study, an injury was defined as an incident that prevented a player from completing a game or practice, or from participating in any future game or practice. This was felt to be a practical definition, although it differs from those used in previous studies. The ideal study of the incidence of injuries would monitor every team during each of their games and practices throughout the season. Since this is impractical, previous studies have taken a longitudinal sample. By contrast, ours took a cross-

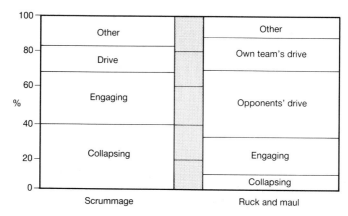

Fig. 2.1 Events leading to injuries occurring in scrums, rucks and mauls.

sectional 'snapshot' view: information was obtained from all the teams playing in Canada during 1 week of a playing season. The data were recorded on a standardized form that was designed with a minimum of free text and reliance on defined responses that could be ticked and the results readily transferred to a computer program.

During the study week, 111 teams participated in 135 games and 224 practices. One hundred injuries were reported; 95 of them occurred during games. A team lost a player to injury once in every 1.4 games and individual players were injured about once a season. Thirteen per cent of injuries occurred during scrums, 23% in rucks and mauls, and 43% were related to tackles.

Of the 13 players injured in the scrums, 10 required medical attention and six players missed subsequent games for an average of 2 weeks. Most of the injuries occurred whilst the scrum was engaging or when it collapsed (Fig. 2.1).

The 25 injuries in rucks and mauls were relatively minor. Only one player required hospital admission, but two-thirds of the injured players missed subsequent games. About 60% of injuries resulted from driving in the ruck and maul by either the opponents or the players' own side. A further quarter occurred as a consequence of collapse and pile-up.

Forty-three players were injured in one or other aspect of tackling (Fig. 2.2). Although most injuries were relatively mild, tackling and being tackled were the major causes of head injuries.

Overall, there were nine fractures of various bones; one player, with complications from a fractured rib, was admitted to hospital. There were 34 joint and ligament injuries, involving (in decreasing order of frequency) the

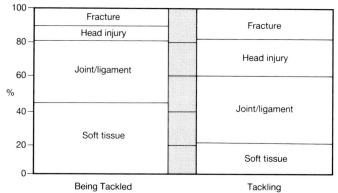

Fig. 2.2 Injuries resulting from tackling and being tackled. Tackling was the most frequent cause of head injury.

shoulder, the ankle and the knee. Half of the players missed further games or practices for an average of 4 weeks.

Of the 11 head injuries, tackling was responsible for seven. Five players required medical attention but none was admitted to hospital. The only two players in the study who lost consciousness sustained their injuries during a tackle-related event; both of these players refrained from playing for the requisite 3 weeks [6]. No significant spinal injuries were reported. Foul play accounted for only three injuries—all the result of illegal tackles.

The current results were compared with the 1988 RFU study (Fig. 2.3)

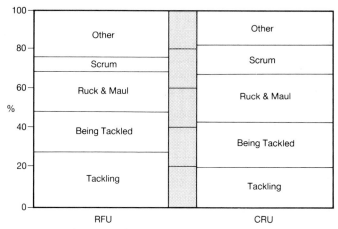

Fig. 2.3 Comparison of patterns of injury in the current Canadian study and in a previous rugby union study. Despite differences in the inclusion criteria, the overall patterns are similar.

[7]

[7]. Although the RFU study included all injuries (even though 47% of the players continued or resumed playing in the game in which they were injured), the phases of play in which injuries occurred were similar, as were injuries according to position. This suggests that a cross-sectional survey provides data which are comparable to the findings of longitudinal studies and may provide a relatively easy means of assessing changes in the patterns of rugby injuries following any modifications of the laws.

Two-thirds of the injuries in rucks and mauls resulted from driving. Experimental Australian law change designed to reduce injuries resulting from this cause have, apparently, not been successful and new experimental laws are being studied. It is important to learn whether such law changes lead to a reduction in these injuries. Although only a relatively small number of injuries resulted from collapse of a ruck or maul, stricter application of the existing law that deals with *wilful* collapse should reduce this cause of injury.

In the scrum, engaging and collapsing are the major hazardous events. Players in other countries who watch games televised from the home countries see that the laws that have been adopted to reduce such injuries are ignored and, unfortunately, follow the example that is set. Laws designed to reduce injuries must be strictly enforced at all levels and in all countries, particularly those that are regarded as setting the example.

Tackling is responsible for a significant proportion of injuries, including some of the most serious [8, 9]. It is difficult to envisage further law changes that could influence tackle-related injuries without altering the fundamental character of the game. An emphasis must, therefore, be placed on coaching this aspect of the game.

Finally, although it is reasonable to assess experimental laws designed to reduce injury in junior players, previous evidence indicates an increasing incidence of injury from the lower to the higher grades [10]. As a consequence, when law changes are demonstrated to reduce the incidence of injury, they should be applied to all levels of the game.

References

1 Burry HC, Calcinai CJ. The need to make rugby safer. *Br Med J* 1988; **1**: 149.
2 Silver JR. The need to make rugby safer. *Br Med J* 1988; **1**: 149–50 (letter).
3 Silver JR. Injury to the spine sustained in rugby. *Br Med J* 1984; **2**: 473.
4 Williams P, McGibbon D. Unstable cervical spine injuries in rugby. *Injury* 1987; **18**: 329–32.
5 Hagerty E. NZ law changes: proven solution to spinal injury. *Rugby* 1986; Sept: 34.
6 International Rugby Football Board Directive. *Concussion* 1985; March.
7 Injuries Working Party. Injuries—4th Report. *Rugby World and Post* 1988; Jan: 7.
8 Silver JR, Gill S. Injuries of the spine sustained during rugby. *Sports Med* 1988; **5**: 328–34.

9 McCoy GF, Piggot J, Macafee A *et al.* Injuries of the cervical spine in schoolboy rugby football. *J Bone Joint Surg* 1984; **66:** 500–3.
10 Myers PT. Injuries presenting from rugby union football. *Med J Aust* 1980; **2:** 17–20.

Discussion

CLARKE: Can I ask to what extent were returns considered absolute?

ENGLAND: The only thing that the Rugby Union would agree to make mandatory was the return of neck injuries. We are hoping, and have tried, to introduce the question of nil returns in order to obtain a more meaningful survey. It's been successful in schools only. With clubs, it doesn't work yet, and I think it is one of the hopeful outcomes of meeting together as rugby physicians and surgeons that we might be able to make an effective and authoritative recommendation to our respective unions that it is mandatory even for selective samples over 5 years, so that we can show trends. I would plead with everyone to persuade their respective unions to analyse figures which are meaningful. The game is a good game; it's a violent game—a collision sport—and it has to be controlled. There is no place for undisciplined violence in the game. But we don't know what we're talking about unless we can get meaningful trend statistics.

BADLEY: One of the advantages of a cross-sectional sample is that you do get compliance. This was achieved apart from one province's returns that were lost in the Canadian post. We had appropriate and 100% returns of the teams who were playing.

ENGLAND: One club secretary used to write in every month. He was superb. But it does depend on the individual. One return was passed to the mini rugby secretary, who decided it wasn't for him and so he put it in the bin. His wife found it as she was throwing out 4 months later, telephoned the secretary of the club and said 'What are we going to do about this?' Believe it or not, he actually got all the returns back.

ETIENNE: I think these are excellent studies but we need a common world-wide system of reporting and analysing injuries. We could then go one step further and try and compare the different series.

ENGLAND: I support Etienne and I think it's something that we really must get our teeth into. There are some members of the International Rugby Board medical advisory sub-committee here, it might be a good idea to make proper moves to obtain an IRB study with proforma based on those already in existence.

GRAYSON: Can I just for my own clarifications make sure I've got what appears to be a very crucially important common denominator between

[9]

Professor Badley and Pat England? Professor Badley said: 'The laws are studiously ignored' and 'The laws are ignored by the same teams through the world' which of course give the corrupting influence on the younger generation as well as those less skilled, and what Pat England's just indicated, that there's nothing wrong with the laws of the game—you've got to be fit and you've got to have the right technique.

Now, if I am correct in my reading, there's a common denominator between Mr England and Professor Badley; there's nothing wrong with the rugby laws so far as professional injury is concerned, it's the operation of the laws and the observance by the referees that is important. If that's correct that's an important domestic fact for me to understand in talking about rugby and the law. I'd just be grateful if I could be affirmed or amended in my own reading of the common denominators I am reading between the two gentlemen.

BADLEY: I agree totally with you. The laws have been changed over several years and evidence suggests that the changes have been beneficial in the reduction of injuries.

ENGLAND: My comment would be that that is too sweeping a statement. I think that the laws as they stand are very good, but as long as there are preventable injuries I very much agree with what everybody advises, that the game should be played according to the laws. The laws are still not yet, in my view, satisfactory.

MOLLOY: The laws certainly have been changed significantly and have helped, but we must resolve the ingenuity of coaching. It is important that coaches be involved in the management of injuries and be capable of dealing with cardiopulmonary resuscitation. Once they have been made aware of the dangers, the risks that they're adding to the game, then perhaps we'll get a more sensible approach.

BURRY: Could I just make one comment on that. I think that Mick is quite correct that the coaches have to be involved and what really is entailed I think is an ethical question. Unfortunately, in New Zealand we have meetings now between coaches and referees at the beginning of the season which are supposed to enable the two groups to get together and to share their knowledge of the game and to ensure the game is refereed according to the spirit of the players so that everybody enjoys it. Unfortunately, what's happened really is that it has given an opportunity for the referees to be intimidated by the senior coaches. A part of the reason we find the laws of the game not being applied by referees is because of the pressure that's applied by the senior players and the senior coaches. Referees quite clearly wish to be well regarded by the players and they try to referee the game according to the way the senior players

want it. The whole paying public see the game being played inappropriately by the senior players and try to mimic it down to school level.
Without the skills they end up damaged.

WALKDEN: The various courses taken by players will always vary. The laws
which have been recommended and brought into operation through
medical recommendations are of no use if we see them being totally
ignored on television. I would think, Professor Badley, that you
mentioned the scrummaging laws, the formation of the scrum and the
prevention of injuries. That particular aspect is one which is being totally
abused and the referee can be intimidated by the domination of some
players.

I can remember when we were first formulating the Medical Digest
supplementing of the International Board, Gordon Rawley, an orthopaedic surgeon to the Welsh Rugby Union, observed before we started
discussing necks again that a motor cyclist would have a 74 times greater
chance of breaking his neck than any player on the field of Cardiff Arms
Park. Sometimes we do have to put this in proportion but as we have said,
and Patrick says in his report, 'one neck a season is one too many.'

3: The Epidemiology of Cervical Injuries in New Zealand

PETER CUNNINGHAM

THE BULK of information presented comes from a study done by the Medical
Sub-committee of the New Zealand Rugby Football Union from 1973 to
1978 [1]. There were 54 cases and as far as possible these were personally
interviewed. They were asked for 60 items of information. Full details were
obtained from 45 (83%), some detail from seven and none from two. The
criteria of a cervical spinal injury were clinical evidence of neurological
damage, radiological evidence of fracture or both. Of the 54 injuries, 25
were serious. There were five deaths (all in 1978), 11 permanent

quadriplegics and nine temporary quadriplegics. The remaining 29 were less serious and some relatively minor. Four of these cases have some residual disability but 36 (60%) made a complete recovery. There was an average of nine cervical spine injuries per year. Assuming that each player has 15 games in a season, and there are 200 000 registered players, the frequency was 1/333 000 games (Table 3.1).

Sixty-two per cent of injuries occurred in players older than 21 years. Of the serious accidents, 50% occurred in those under 21 and of these 50% were under 17. Injuries were distributed throughout the whole season, but occurred more frequently in the third quarter of games. Fourteen per cent occurred in schoolboy rugby but the majority were in club competition (Table 3.2). Forwards were affected in 68% of all injuries and 52% involved the front row. The hooker seemed to be the player most at risk. Just over half of the injuries occurred in the scrum phase of the game. The majority of these were associated with some form of collapse but in some instances, necks were broken before the collapse occurred (Table 3.3).

In six accidents, players had difficulty forming the front row. Five of these led to quadriplegia or death. Nineteen injuries occurred during tackles with the tackled person being at greater risk.

Comments from injured players included the following: the front rows stand too close, with feet forward, making it difficult to form the scrum; locks and back rows may apply pressure before the front row has properly formed; half-backs may place the ball in the scrum and the weight is applied before the front row has properly formed. All six props injured in scrums were under the age of 20. Lack of awareness of potential dangers was prevalent in this survey. Inexperience was probably a factor in three instances but there was no direct evidence of disproportion in size or weight.

Recommendations

1 All players should perform exercises especially designed to strengthen the muscles of the neck and shoulder girdles.

Table 3.1 Frequency of injury in relation to player/games

Number of players	200 000
Average number of games/ season	15 in 3 000 000 exposures
Average number of injuries/ season	9
Average number of injuries/ player/game	1 in 333 000

Table 3.2 Type of game ($n=42$)

School	Club competition	Training and trials	Social
6–14.2%	22–52.3%	6–14.2%	8–19%

Table 3.3 Playing position/injury

	Prop	Hooker	Lock	Back row		Total
Forwards	13	11	2	5		31
Injured in scrums	6	9	—	1		16
Injured in other play	7	2	2	4		15
	Half	Five-eighth	Three-quarter	Wing	Full-back	
Backs	2	4	1	4	3	14

2 Front rows of opposing scrums should be properly formed before the locks and back rows join the scrum.

3 The referee should ensure that the ball is not put into the scrum before the scrum is properly formed and with all players adequately bound.

4 Players, coaches and referees must be made aware of the danger of charging blindly into rucks and mauls with the neck flexed.

5 Players at risk should adopt a position which protects the neck. In New Zealand, body position is taught to younger players especially by asking them to shorten their necks by hunching their shoulders, to extend the neck slightly and to hollow the lumbar spine, and adopting the 'eyeball to eyeball and spine in line' position.

In New Zealand, some adjustments have been made to the domestic rules to protect young players. These rules go up to but exclude senior reserves. They include the following: (a) the scrum cannot rotate past 45°; (b) the half-back cannot pass through the mid-line of the scrum; (c) the scrum can only progress up to 1.5 m; and (d) in forming a scrum, players must come a metre apart, touch and then engage.

The scrum numbers are dictated by the attacking team. If the attacking team decides to pull off a number 8, the other side must pull off a number 8. A player who is sent off is replaced by one experienced in that position.

The Orthopaedic Association in New Zealand has been approached by the

New Zealand Rugby Football Union Advisory Committee to notify all neck injuries to the New Zealand Union, so that a register of neck injuries can be ascertained. The more accurate the figures we obtain, the easier it will be to make recommendations.

Two illustrative cases

1 Scott, a 17-year-old seventh former, was injured in a practice when two opposing scrums stood apart and forcefully engaged. He was in the front row when his head hit the opposing player's head or shoulder and was forced into hyperflexion. He was immediately quadriplegic. On admission X-rays revealed a complete bilateral facet dislocation of C4 on C5 and he was noted to have a C5 quadriplegia.

He was taken to theatre that day and under local anaesthetic, skull tongs were applied and then under general anaesthetic he was intubated. Closed reduction of the dislocation was confirmed by X-ray. Subsequently his general condition deteriorated and 2 days later he died from respiratory arrest. This injury was totally preventable.

2 Sam aged 13 was playing number 8 for his school. He ran around the side of the scrum and was tackled. He was still clutching the ball with both arms and fell forward on to the back of his head (flexed) and then the opposing forwards fell on top of him. He heard and felt a crack in his neck and then lost feeling and movement in all limbs. He was left lying prone in the mud with his head flexed and rotated. I attended from the sideline and was confronted with a situation I hoped would never present. As his neck was in such a bizarre position and because Sam was complaining of discomfort I protected his neck while he was turned onto his back. I then applied gentle traction and rotation to his head until it easily came back to a near neutral position. He was then supported until the ambulance arrived some 10–15 minutes later. At this stage Sam started to move his feet and then hands. By the time he was on a cervical stretcher he had reasonable movement of all limbs.

On admission to hospital he was found to have a partial C4 cord lesion. X-rays revealed the presence of a unilateral facet dislocation at C2–C3 which reduced after the application of skeletal traction over several hours. Over the next few days his neurological status improved, but not completely. It was decided to stabilise the C2–C3 level. At operation it was found there had been soft tissue injury and spinal fusion was performed. He subsequently made a good recovery and was discharged with a residual C5–C6 deficit, but improving.

This injury at this age was unusual. The point for discussion is, if and when one is justified in moving a neck as first aid.

Discussion

McLATCHIE: Can I make a comment on the movement of players with neck injuries? The thinking has always been to apply traction to the neck of the player on the basis that if there is a fracture it should be reduced. More recently, we've been worried that a C1–C2 lesion may be made worse. Hyper-extension injury of the neck may occur, similar to judicial hanging. In those situations we would suggest that traction should not be applied. The other thing I would like to say is that Piggot and Gordon wrote a letter suggesting that these players should be log-rolled: that prognosis was better for the neck injured player if there was a doctor present, and they used several examples of how these players were moved.

MOLLOY: A problem with neck injury, especially a high cervical lesion is difficult breathing and determining whether it is due to the intensity of competition or serious spinal cord injury. I have one experience of an international player who was injured. As we took him off he didn't have a serious injury—he could move his hands and legs—but he did hear a crack in his neck. He turned to the two medical people dealing with him and said: 'I hope you get it right because I'll sue you otherwise'. He was actually a lawyer and he was joking, of course, but I think it emphasises the responsibilities we have in that situation. Probably the most important thing is to have the right equipment available. In that area I find a scoop orthopaedic stretcher extremely helpful, because it's very rare you have enough people to help in that situation with a bad neck injury.

GRAYSON: Yes, only I am fascinated on that very point because I was going to ask Dr Cunningham a question and make a comment. The question is this: to what extent do your revelations, your research and your teaching go to trying to educate the referees and the coaches of those levels who are not fully, as it were, experienced? We know that George Crawford, the famous metropolitan police superintendent abandoned and walked off the field when Bristol played Newport because he said: 'I spend Monday to Friday nicking villains and I don't want to do it on Saturday afternoon!'

The point is that if in fact the schoolmaster who is trained, perhaps has a part-time coaching facility and the referee who does it as a bit of fun but has stopped playing, unless they are given some guidance you've got a great lacuna. The other interesting point is this: I'm very much involved because of course of my origins as it were with the association football world and only a few weeks ago I was at Lilleshall addressing the FA, the doctors and so forth and John O'Hara, who is the chairman of the FA Medical Committee has told me how he is doing his best to integrate the St

John's ambulance people into sports medicine as a first base. I come back to the comment about the need to educate, and also the question.

Just in parentheses, I remember this was in the *Daily Telegraph*, the Bath captain was injured, with a neck injury, and I remember because I had a case concerning a soldier at this time and I wanted to know what had happened at Bath. Dr Ian Granderson, who is the Bath doctor, used the very facility which you have just told us—he kept the player mobile and sent for the ambulance and the retraction and the scoop facility was available. The scoop facility is *not* available at school level, and is not available at every club level—what do you do, apart from educating those who are doing paramedical activities? So my comment is a general one, but the question is: how far have you gone in trying to educate these people who've got such a responsibility?

CUNNINGHAM: The referees do a first aid course and they are aware of potential dangers. We may overlook coaches in our preventative medicine although we have schools in New Zealand for junior coaches and a big part consists of safety. The St John's Ambulance Brigade is having difficulty recruiting members and a large number of games don't have the presence of a St John's Ambulance member.

HUGO: I think if you have got a doctor present so much the better. There is one problem that we've talked about and I think it is our biggest problem, namely the first aider. I just wanted to add something that we've managed to make the rugby authority accept: that no rugby can take place unless there is a qualified first aider and minimum first aid equipment. In Japan or Argentina they do not play rugby unless they've got a doctor there. So, in my view, no trained first aider, no minimum equipment; no rugby.

WALKDEN: That gets a very crucial point across; the larger the number of games being played in the country, the more difficult that is. In the introductive league rugby in the Rugby Football Union it has happened now that the referee has refused to start a game even at the area level because there was not a doctor present—but actually there he was applying the laws wrongly: the requirement is for a person with nursing or medical experience. The more games are played in the country, the more difficult of course it is to apply that. We have recommended for 20 years that people should attend first aid courses.

EAVES: It's perhaps appropriate here to raise an initiative which we took with the Hampshire Football Association, and St John's Ambulance, a 3-hour resuscitation and emergency first aid course was set up. From 1991 it will be mandatory for any team affiliated to the Hampshire FA to have at least one person with that qualification, renewable every 3 years. It is a subsidised course which costs £10 and a third of all clubs have sent a player into the scheme.

MacAig: I think there should be no attempt at all to reduce cervical injuries on the field. Those who have experience of closed reduction even in theatre have difficulty. We're all taught to flex and rotate the head and bring it back to neutral and there's no 'pop' to be heard or felt. On the field this should not be attempted. Rotating the head to neutral? Most of the severe injuries are unifacet dislocations and rotating the head doesn't reduce it and I think we should, on the field at least, stabilise, not apply traction, which in my mind means pulling the head. Without defining injury we should leave well alone, treat it as very unstable and get them to a hospital.

We have a lot of GPs throughout the world who X-ray patients and rely on a radiologist's report. In most places I've worked, radiologists really have problems reporting on necks and heads and if there is any doubt of a serious injury the X-ray should be seen by an orthopaedic surgeon and the proper X-rays requested.

Walkden: Skill in any game is uncoachable but technique certainly is, such as the technique of tackling and of being tackled. The prevention aspects of the recommendations made by the New Zealand Rugby Football Union were discussed by the Rugby Football Union and accepted and recommended to the International Board, who accepted measures to stabilise the scrum, except for the back foot and the 1.5 metre rule. This rejection of our recommendations is something about which we should feel more strongly because injury prevention should receive absolute priority.

Three months after the last meeting of the Medical Advisory Sub-committee of the International Board in 1988, a hooker's neck was broken following a pushover scrum and resulted in quadriplegia.

England: I'm interested in the number of serious injuries in New Zealand each year because our experience is not as big as that, even though we have over 3000 rugby playing units under the jurisdiction of the Rugby Football Union. To come to the point made by Etienne Hugo, it's very difficult to provide a doctor for every venue, especially if you don't realise that there are other sports claiming doctors as well and there simply aren't enough. I think there is a greater case for training paramedics, training volunteers so that they are 'skilled' so they know precisely what's going on. I think there would be a case then for making it mandatory to have somebody who had passed a sensible, recognised course in paramedical skills to be present if there is no doctor available.

Davies: We have people from all over the world here, asking them what is happening in various countries. In Wales, we have an association called the Welsh Association of Sports Trainers. These are lay people and they attend courses and they're given a certificate of confidence and attendance in sports first aid.

References
1 Medical Advisory Committee of NZ RFU. *Study on cervical spine injuries*, 1978.

4: Severe Spinal Injuries due to Rugby in South Africa

ETIENNE P.HUGO

VARIOUS epidemiological studies on spinal injuries in rugby have been conducted in South Africa. The results in one study on the incidence of various injuries at all levels of the game and one on severe spinal injuries are reported [1].

1824 rugby injuries occurring between 1975 and 1984 were analysed in Pretoria. All these injuries occurred at the main rugby stadium and all players were affiliated to the South African Rugby Board which in turn is affiliated to the International Rugby Football Board.

In the initial study, head and neck injuries were grouped together. 773 (42.4%) of the injuries involved these areas. Closer scrutiny however indicated that only 45 (2.5%) were neck injuries.

All these injuries were musculoligamentous and no neurological deficit was reported. None of these cases required surgery.

Catastrophic spinal injuries associated with severe neurological deficit always cause greater interest and concern. All these severe injuries are treated in two spinal injury units in South Africa. Most of the injuries were admitted to the Cape Town Unit. During the period 1963–89, 105 patients were treated there. The patients' records of 76 were reviewed and 52 of these were followed up.

The mechanisms of injuries were compared with those reported in other series [2–5] (Table 4.1). Silver conducted his study in England, Taylor and

Table 4.1 Mechanisms of injury—international study

Reference	Dates	Scrum	Ruck/maul	Tackle Ball carrier	Tackle Tackler	Foul	Line out	Other open	Total
Silver [2]	1952–82								
Forwards		13	14	3	4	2	0		55
Backs			4	9	6	0	0		37
Taylor & Coolican [3]	1960–85	62%	14%	22%				2%	37
Williams & McKibbin [4]	1964–84	12	9	6	3				30
Kew [5]	1963–89								
Forwards		15	10	8	6	2	1		42
Backs		0	5	16	13	0	0		34

Table 4.2 Further analysis of the Cape Town injuries series (1963–88)

Position	Scrum (%)	Ruck/ maul (%)	Ball carrier (%)	Tackler (%)	Foul play (%)	Total (%)
Front row	17.2	5.2	4.0	0	1.3	27.6
Forwards	2.6	7.9	6.0	7.9	1.3	27.6
Half-backs	0	4.0	6.6	1.3	0	11.8
Back-line	0	2.6	14.5	15·8	0	32.9

Table 4.3 Details of play in the scrum at the time of injury [3]

Mechanism	Schoolboys	Adults
Engagement	4	11
Collapse	2	2
Push after collapse	1	2
Popped up	1	0
Late push	0	0
Total	8	15

Table 4.4 Details of playing position amongst players from three countries with neck injuries

Position	Wales 1984	Australia 1987	Cape Town 1989	
Hooker	3	16	14	
Prop	10	14	7	
Forwards	9	4	21	
Flank	(5)			(6)
Lock	(4)			(10)
No. 8				(5)
Back-line	7	3	34	
Full-back				(3)
Centre	(4)			(14)
Fly-half	(2)			(6)
Wing				(8)
Scrum-half	(1)			(3)
Total	29	37	76	

Coolican in Australia, and Kew in Cape Town, South Africa. Williams and McKibban's study was conducted in Wales on behalf of the IRFB (Table 4.2). 27.6% of these injuries occurred in the front row players and the same number in other forwards. The tackle was responsible for the greatest number of injuries (54·7%), and scrums together with ruck and maul for 19.75%. Taylor and Coolican analysed the scrum in more detail. The engagement phase was identified as the most important facet of play in those cases responsible for injuries. 15 in a series of 23 injuries were reported here (Table 4.3). Front row forwards were more prone to injuries.

More back-line players were reported injured in the Cape Team series than those in Wales and Australia (34 out of a total of 76 injuries) (Table 4.4). The 76 players sustaining severe spinal injuries in the Cape Town study were analysed according to age. 28 were under 21 years and 41 over this age. 30.8% of the injuries occurred at schoolboy level.

The total number of severe spinal injuries due to rugby are still unacceptably high in South Africa: 11 occurred in 1984 and 1985, nine in 1986, 10 in 1987, 12 in 1988, and 13 in 1989 [6]. Statistics are unfortunately not available world-wide. The South African experience does not compare too unfavourably with those in other rugby playing countries when one considers that more than 300 000 rugby players are affiliated to the South African Rugby Board alone. An unknown number of rugby players are however not affiliated to this Board.

When scrutinizing these injuries it was noted that 28.2% of the severe injuries occurred amongst South African Rugby Board players.

Conclusion

In the study of 1824 rugby injuries the incidence of neck injuries was very low (2.5%). No neurological deficit occurred in any of these cases.

In the study of severe spinal injuries the incidence of these injuries was lower (28.2%) under players affiliated to the South African Rugby Board and playing under well-controlled conditions than those playing without this control.

A definite tendency towards more back-line players sustaining severe spinal injuries are recorded.

References

1 Wessels LGD. *Report on the incidence of rugby players in Pretoria, South Africa*, presented to the Northern Transvaal Rugby Union 1985. (Report not published.)
2 Silver JR. Injuries of the spine sustained in rugby. *Br Med J* 1984; **147**: 112–18.
3 Taylor TKF, Coolican MRJ. Spinal-cord injuries in Australian footballers 1960–1985. *Med J Aust* 1984; **147**: 112.

4 Williams P, McKibbin B. *Unstable cervical spine injuries in rugby: A 20 year review.* Report to IRFB.

5 Kew TG. *Catastrophic neck injuries in rugby.* University of Cape Town, South Africa (Thesis).

6 Hugo EP. *Report on the incidence of severe spinal injuries in South African Rugby 1990,* presented to the South African Rugby Board. (Report not published.)

PART 2
SPECIFIC INJURIES AND
THEIR ASSESSMENT

5: The Field Assessment of Rugby Injuries

JOHN CHASE

IT IS difficult to educate the American public about what rugby is; it is an amateur sport which means no money and no money means no press. Many parents think it is a dangerous sport and it is difficult for them to believe that it is not when they see lacerations and blood. Another problem is litigation and the temptation after an injury to ask: 'Who am I going to sue?' A serious injury in a rugby game on a field with potholes, without an administrator and with a referee who is a retired player could invite law suits and a subsequent reluctance to make ground available. At college level the game is not administrated with the same authority as other sports and so players may misbehave. Under age drinking is an acknowledged problem with rugby players in the USA and that further alienates administration and officials.

In the USA there are more than 50 doctors involved in rugby medicine and in touring with teams. Some who have been players have difficulty making the transition from player to administrator and doctor. At training camps for USA national players, they are examined and an injury history obtained. It will probably never be possible to have a doctor at every match and a competent referee may not be available. At least one person on every team should be responsible for the medical kit, the first-aid bag, and have training in first aid and resuscitation. Referees should ensure these requirements before each game. All referees would benefit from first aid and resuscitation training.

Studies of American rugby players indicate that approximately one in 10 will be badly enough injured in the season to miss at least one match. This compared favourably with a 50% incidence of injury in American grid iron football for players over a season [1]. We believe the lower incidence of injuries in rugby football is due to the absence of blocking and protective equipment. The provision of medical care at rugby pitches in the USA has been primitive compared with European and Pacific countries. Commonly, no medical or paramedical person is present at a match, the vast majority of teams do not have a trainer or a person qualified in first aid nor in emergency treatment or recognition of injury.

Players who are seriously injured, or at risk of additional injury, should not be allowed to play until they have been evaluated, treated and recovered completely. Players with contagious conditions, such as scrum rash, should not be allowed to play. Open or bleeding wounds must be covered; referees should evaluate teams and players for health problems and injuries prior to matches.

A particular area of concern is preventing the injured player from resuming participation too soon. This is *vital* when a head injury or concussion has been suffered. The player must not be allowed to resume until he has been medically evaluated, fully recovered and the 3 weeks designated by law should have elapsed before he returns to competition.

It is important to keep accurate records and obtain informed consent for treatment. When injuries cannot be handled at the field, support facilities of ambulance and paramedical services can often be obtained at low cost as a public service and as an enjoyable afternoon or weekend for individuals who would otherwise be on call at home or at some other site.

It is important to have people immediately or rapidly available, who can help to transport an injured player, especially when a spinal injury has occurred. Stretchers which can be assembled around a patient are valuable in moving an injured player who cannot be picked up from the ground without support. Whenever there is a question of spinal injury, trained people should be the only ones to move the patient.

The most important thing for those involved with the recognition and care of injuries is to be prepared. There must be transportation and communication available to transport an injured player to a hospital emergency room or to call paramedics and ambulance services if necessary. Car keys should be in a known location and with a designated person. The vehicle and the keys must be determined before the match. The closest hospital or emergency room should be located and contacted to inform them that rugby players may be seen in their facility or they may be called to treat an injury. The location of the nearest telephone should be identified so that communication can be carried out when necessary. The phone number of the local ambulance service and/or the hospital should also be known before the match has begun. Coins should be available in the trainer's kit so that a telephone call can be made with the minimum of difficulty and confusion.

Players should be inspected and counselled always to wear a mouth guard and not chew gum. Projections such as buckles, rings or watches should not be allowed and players should not wear necklaces. Shinguards are particularly recommended for the front row and a single stud at the toe in the boot is prohibited.

Players with open wounds that cannot easily be covered or repaired should not be permitted to continue playing. Players should have vaccinations and current tetanus prophylaxis. Whenever more than emergency treatment is required, the patient should be referred for appropriate medical care.

There are many materials which can be placed in the medical kit: Vaseline and heat ointments, septic spray, spray or powder for athletes' foot, adherents for taping and strapping and cold sprays may also be of value. Remember that the medical kit should be adapted to the needs, knowledge and experience of those using it. Elastic tape or Elastoplast of various sizes can be very helpful in strapping knees and elbows. Ordinary athletic tape in the 2.5 and 5 cm size are stocked with dressings which can be used under the taping. Paper tape is good for applying dressings and holding them in place.

Antibiotics, cleats and a stud wrench, contact lens holders and a positive pressure breathing mask with a one-way valve may be included. An eye wash cup is helpful to clean mud from the eye and help with contact lenses. Vaseline impregnated dressing can be used to pad Achilles tendon areas and other prominences.

Instruments such as toe-nail clippers, scissors, scalpels and other tools for treating wounds and applying dressings are useful. Syringes, needles, sutures and appropriate anaesthetics should be placed in the case which can be used in the repair of lacerations. Tongue blades are used to apply Vaseline and antibiotics and depress the tongue.

Non-sterile gauze pads are of value in many situations. Padded adherent materials that can be placed over tender areas and a triangular bandage or sling for fractures is invaluable.

Medications such as muscle relaxants, anti-inflammatories, aspirin and sun screen can be added. Electrical tape is also very popular for covering the ears and keeping them tied to the head to prevent cauliflower ear in scrums and rucks. A large thermos can be used to hold ice or ice bags. The latter are easily made by placing ice in a zip lock bag and a large fluid container can be used to fill squeeze bottles which are made available at the ground.

The incidence and type of injury as well as how they relate to players in certain phases of the game have been studied. A recent Welsh survey indicated that 22% of injuries occur to the upper limbs, 29% to the head. Most common are lacerations and contusions; 4% involved the neck and may be catastrophic; and 33% of the injuries are to the lower limbs [2] (Fig. 5.1).

A trainer must teach himself to watch the action on the field, look for an injury about to occur and identify one that has occurred. He must listen for cries of help or assistance. He must understand the mechanisms of injury; this is the most important thing that he can do to help him to be aware as he runs onto the field, for it will allow him to know what sort of problem he

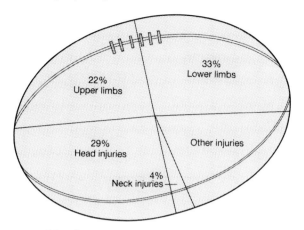

Fig. 5.1 Summary of distribution of injuries according to Richards [2].

may encounter when he arrives. Preparation will improve his ability to recognise and treat injury; a trainer must be familiar with the types of injuries and the dangers of certain phases of the game. Scrums are known to be a dangerous phase of the game and in particular the collision of the two packs coming together. This can generate tons of force and can be the site of injuries to the head, neck, shoulders and other parts of the body.

The International Rugby Football Board has studied the scrum in an attempt to make it safer. Variations in binding of the front row, or first five, as well as limited wheeling of the scrum and limited time that the ball may be kept in the back of the scrum without coming out, have all been tried with no results.

The most dangerous incident in the game has often been thought to be the collapsed scrum. In fact, statistics have shown that collision in the front row and the damage sustained in tackles are more dangerous. Nevertheless, collapsing of the scrum is a place where necks may be broken. Popping up of the hooker is a third dangerous area that should be made illegal. Tackles are the most dangerous phase of the game with slightly more injuries to the tackler than to the tackled player. Correct methods of tackling must be taught by coaches to avoid injury. Players must be taught to fall in such a way as to avoid injury and the tackler should learn to put his head behind the tackled player, while the tackled player should learn to turn his body to present a less vulnerable target. In New Zealand, martial arts techniques are taught to players to teach them how to fall correctly. In spite of all coaching and teaching, injuries will occur during the tackle phase of the game and the trainer will often be called on to treat them.

Foul play accounts for 7–10% of injury in rugby and must not be allowed in a game that is already physical enough. Techniques of physical intimidation and foul play should not be allowed. Players should not be permitted to stay on the pitch after they have been warned and/or performed a dangerous act towards another player. Kicking and punching must not be allowed. Foul play must be penalised severely. Rucks, mauls and pile-ups also create sites for injury. The frequent disorganisation of these phases of the game often predispose to an accident. Players should be taught not to dive over the ball or fall on players. They must protect their necks and they should turn their bodies to avoid unnecessary or dangerous contact. They should learn to enter rucks and mauls with care and protect themselves in all phases of the game. Trainers should keep their eyes on the match at all times to determine when an injury occurs and be ready to go on the field when necessary.

Line-outs are associated with injuries to the head, shoulders and neck as well as the legs. Jumping brings many players into contact and foul play may also occur. The kicking phase of the game is also dangerous, both to the approaching player and to the person who has kicked the ball. Illegal playing of the man after he is rid of the ball should be disallowed and players should learn to protect themselves in situations when they may be kicked or when their leg may be struck.

One of the most common areas of injury is to the joints, ligaments and other associated structures. A trainer must assess the player for swelling, joint tenderness or laxity of ligaments. The opposite side can be used for comparison to determine how much is normal and how much is due to the injury. An assessment must be made whether the player can remain in the match with or without appropriate strapping or must come to the sidelines for further evaluation and treatment.

Remember the eponym 'ICE' which stands for ice, compression and elevation. These are important for minimising the injury and speeding recovery. Weight bearing should be limited whenever there is suspicion of a significant problem and medical evaluation and appropriate X-rays obtained when necessary.

One of the most serious and many times underdiagnosed and treated injuries in rugby are those to the head. Players should be carefully evaluated for loss of consciousness, amnesia and mental or physical dysfunction. A concussion is an impairment of neural functioning and may involve loss of consciousness. A first degree, grade 1 or mild concussion may involve no loss of consciousness; a second degree, grade 2 or moderate injury, may be associated with 5 minutes or less of loss of consciousness; and a severe, or grade 3 injury, with more than 5 minutes of unconsciousness. Players may also have amnesia or loss of memory for events leading up to or immediately after the event; they may be impaired in their ability to ambulate or perform simple mental functions such as counting backwards by sevens. Whenever there is a question of a significant concussion, the player must not be allowed to continue in the match and this must be understood and agreed upon by the referee, the captain, the coach and the player himself. The trainer, first aid person or doctor's decision in this regard must be final and unassailable.

Another area of injury, often seen on the rugby field, is fractures and dislocations. It is important to determine if deformity is present or whether there is significant swelling. Is there false motion or movement where there should be none? Is crepitation, grinding or crunching present in a limb to suggest a bony fracture? Is a joint particularly painful, restricted in movement or deformed, such as where a dislocation may be present? Rapid evaluation and treatment of these injuries is often extremely helpful. When there is question of a fracture or dislocation, early reduction is permissible if excessive force is not required and the patient does not suffer too much pain. Medical attention is necessary following these injuries. Cramps may also occur. These may be associated with lack of hydration, inadequate water intake, electrolyte depletions, such as salt, potassium or magnesium, and they may occur with fatigue or other problems. Counter-irritation and stretching are effective methods of relieving a cramp. Stretching the opposite limb or the affected limb or pinching the upper lip below the nose can often relieve this painful situation.

Contusions are very frequent in rugby and they may be treated with the classical method, the time honoured magic sponge, ice water or the more modern techniques of ethylchloride may be utilised. This material gives a local freezing of the skin over the injured part and is a form of counter-irritation.

Many injuries on the rugby field can be treated immediately and allow the player to continue. Some injuries however will not lend themselves to on-the-field treatment and the player must be treated off the field, either at the local emergency facility or in the hospital.

A captain and the coach must decide whether this length of time is permissible or if the team plays short. It is in the best interest of the doctor and the player to hurry the repair and allow a return to competition. It helps to have a supporting hand and caring person at the rugby field when injuries occur. We must demand that players have adequate health and disability insurance coverage. Field treatment for free will not always be available and many health professions are not willing to treat patients in this situation of less than perfect conditions. Nonetheless, players plus medical care equals a safer game.

Discussion

JONES: I'm a medical officer for the Welsh under 19s side. I'd like to thank you for the point that you raised about having referees first aid qualified. Those of you who passed a referee's exam, as I did many years ago, realise how arduous it is. We could introduce a simple first aid exam to go with it.

PAYNE: It's unfortunate but I was not surprised to hear that rugby in America is at risk of being strangled at birth by litigation. Both doctors and administrators could incur negligence. There is no particular precedent and one has to refer to other potential sources of law such as legislation and decided cases in civil law. In the absence of those, we have to look to other potential sources, namely textbooks and experts' opinion. This conference has many experts and carries weighty authority. The published proceedings should be disseminated and sent to those authorities you're wishing to influence.

WALKDEN: Every now and then I wander through the parks and the recreation grounds of England and see how the games are carrying on there and still the anachronism of the bucket and sponge is the only equipment they have.

References

1 Micheli LJ, Riseborough E. Incidence of injuries in rugby. *J Sports Med* 1986; **22**: 69–73.
2 Richards H. *A Review of Rugby Injuries*. IRFB Congress on Rugby Injuries, Oxfordshire, 1986.

6: Evaluating Spinal Injuries

MICK MOLLOY

THE STRUCTURES in the spine—the vertebrae; the discs; the nervous tissue; the muscles and ligaments may all be sites of injury. In the lumbar area the risks are less than in the cervical area. A patient in the clinic who plays rugby is likely to have one of the problems which also afflict non-players. It is important to remember all the possibilities. For example, there is the occasional player who uses back pain as an excuse for not playing. If one looks at rugby it is not surprising that this occasionally happens, and although it can happen at any level of the game, it is more likely in the less-skilled player.

There are various ways of examining the lumbar spine. Chest expansion measurement should be included because underlying ankylosing spondylitis is a condition that should exclude players from rugby and spinal stiffness with limited chest expansion may suggest this possibility.

As a general rule, rheumatologists tend to talk about lower lumbar disc lesions as the commonest cause of back pain and a quick way of examining the patient is to get them to walk on their toes. This will show whether subjects have a weakness of the S1 root. Walking on the heels will show whether they have a weakness in L5.

Whether an X-ray should be included is open to question. How one interprets the X-ray in relation to the sport is even more controversial. A patient with Schmorl's nodes, with a history of back pain raises the question of whether they should actually play rugby or not. Pathologically, a Schmorl's node is a vertical subluxation of the disc through the vertebral end-plate, i.e. a fracture of the vertebral end-plate. It is a pathological problem which one sees in young people who are of the rugby playing age, so we have to take a decision. If symptoms are not severe they should be allowed to play.

A patient may have severe back pain and drop-foot due to a disc prolapse and be considered for surgery. Such cases may resume playing and thus prove that there is no requirement for surgery. These patients are plentiful. When a disc protrusion is demonstrated radiologically, should one treat the patient or the X-ray? At a recent conference on back pain, somebody quoted a paper on back pain and computerised tomography (CT). One group were patients who had CT scans of the lumbar spine and symptoms of sciatica, the other were age-related controls. The radiologists were asked to give their comments on the findings and on the possible clinical outcome. The patients who had no symptoms scored higher than the patients with symptoms, illustrating how selective one has to be in requesting such investigations and how carefully one must evaluate them, because X-ray changes do not necessarily relate to the patient's symptoms. X-ray evidence of osteoarthritis in the spine does not mean a player has to stop.

Will rugby increase the risk of neck and back osteoarthritis (spondylosis)? There is a suspicion that it does. Most forwards in rugby seem to have cervical spondylosis. Schauermann's disease, a form of osteochondritis of the vertebral edge, occurs in young people and is frequently asymptomatic. When found in a young player one has to decide whether or not he should go on. Often it is found in players who have incidental X-rays done later in life who have been playing rugby at a high level without any symptoms, so

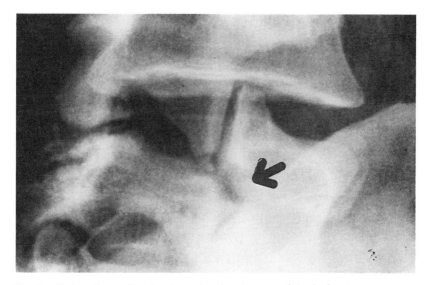

Fig. 6.1 Oblique X-ray of the lumbar spine showing a crack in the lamina (spondylolysis).

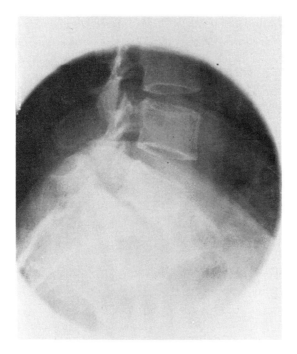

Fig. 6.2 X-ray of the spine showing slippage of one vertebrae as a consequence of spondylolysis.

it is a difficult decision. In most of these, some disc space narrowing will be apparent. So the potential for developing symptoms exists. A defect in the spinal arch (spondylolysis) is another X-ray abnormality which can concern us (Fig. 6.1). If there is associated slippage, whether or not to allow a player to perform is a delicate question (Fig. 6.2). If it is an incidental finding and there is no back pain we tend to let them play. However, there is uncertainty about whether this is a correct decision.

A condition that is seen with regularity in those with stiffness is ankylosing spondylitis or spondarthritis. It is important to ask for a family history of back pain and to look for evidence of psoriasis because this may be associated with spondylitis in the absence of peripheral arthritis. In a rugby context it is necessary to ask for a history of sexual activity. An episode of non-specific urethritis may subsequently lead to recurrent inflammation of tendon or ligament attachments (enthesopathies) as well as sacroiliitis. One needs to look for unilateral sacroiliitis. Bone scans may be used but are not particularly helpful. CT scans can show early erosive changes.

The cervical spine is of particular importance and one must teach the need for keeping the neck slightly flexed, or in a good anatomical position for tackling and for hitting rucks and mauls. It is important because of the anatomy of the cervical spine. When the neck is slightly flexed at 30°, it becomes one unit, it straightens and loses its lordotic curve, so that when the head makes contact with an opponent, the cervical spine is compressed between the opponent and the body. Most injuries occur in flexion. Studies have examined pressure areas using laboratory models. Keeping the head up in tackles and when going into rucks is important. For the front row forward who is just about to make contact in the scrum, this may not be a realistic goal. One common problem in the neck is impingement neuropathies. Patients, having made contact during a game develop sharp pain in the neck, shoulder and down the arm, with or without tingling in the fingers and sometimes with weakness. These patients usually do not have any restriction of neck movement. Frequently they are ignored. When acute, the symptoms are worrying but in most cases they improve although they may be associated with weakness which indicates neuropraxia. These cases must leave the field and be evaluated carefully. Mild cases improve and sometimes even the more severe examples will also recover very quickly. Some unfortunately go on to develop significant weakness. In my experience of 15–20 young players in a university setting, all made a full recovery and returned to play rugby. If there is underlying cervical spondylosis then recurrence of symptoms is problematic and in these, a return to rugby is less certain.

Under this category is the acute anterior spine syndrome, first described by Schneider. After contact, the player hits the ground and has no feeling in the arms or legs, but tends to retain posterior column sensation. He recovers rapidly but the symptoms indicate how severely the spine has been injured in the accident.

The next group is the acute cervical sprain and this is the commonest problem. It is frequent in all age groups. Dealing with a national squad of 25 players one will have at least a dozen a year. Some have to cease rugby for weeks. Some of them have to drop out for longer, and occasionally do so for good. However, most of them do well. It tends to be a recurrent problem and one has to talk to the coach and go into detail about technique in tackling or scrummaging. It is impossible to avoid these injuries in a sport like rugby. They have to be taken seriously but, as with neuropraxia they tend to improve.

An X-ray of the neck is necessary and one has to make the investigation request specific. Flexion-extension and odontoid views ensure that there is no higher cervical damage. Management includes collars and anti-inflammatory drugs, rest, physiotherapy and careful evaluation to make sure there is no late onset neurological problem. It may be associated with mild concussion. Longitudinal studies are necessary to determine if these injuries predispose to long-term symptoms.

An acute cervical disc lesion produces an acutely painful neck, similar to a lumbar disc protrusion but more severe. This is not too difficult to diagnose because the patient is unable to do anything—even rest. It requires strong analgesia, a collar and sometimes traction in hospital. If there is associated weakness in any of the nerve roots then there may be a need for urgent treatment in hospital. Most improve. If surgery is necessary affected players tend not to resume the sport. For the patient with a suspected serious neck injury, maintaining the airway is vital. At international level an anaesthetist is available in case of difficulty. That anaesthetist has a special call code to arrive on the pitch. Frequently, a neck-injured player is lying on his face. Once an airway is established and the patient is breathing and there is not a high cervical lesion, it is safe to apply slight traction. It requires four other people to turn the patient, using a spinal stretcher. The person holding the head must be in charge and tell the other people when to do things, whilst keeping on traction and watching the patient's respiration and pulse. The patient can then be placed on the stretcher which may be simple—an ordinary door will do. When examining breathing difficulties, interpretation of dyspnoea can be problematic because patients have been running around the pitch. In one example, the patient was able to say that he could not breath and an emergency tracheotomy was done half an hour later in hospital.

In Ireland the rugby playing population is about 30 000 and is similar to Wales or Scotland. Over 12 years experience most cord injuries who survived are alive. Two have died. Survivors are now leading reasonable lives, with restriction. Some are married. All have jobs and have adapted their homes and environment and have received help from the rugby clubs they belonged to, or the Rugby Union. Every Christmas, they are given a special bonus; they can go to all the internationals if they wish, in a secluded area in the stand. For the last 2 years there have been no such injuries in Ireland.

Possible ways of reducing the incidence of these devastating injuries include selecting players of the right stature to suit their positions and explaining the risk to coaches, referees and players. Unfortunately players do not take a lot of notice of medical people talking to them about injury. One suggestion is that a select group of international players should be asked to make a film explaining how they protected themselves; how they experienced and coped with these risks over the years. Strength is important and neck exercises are essential. Skill and technique are critical. Learning to stay on the feet all the time is essential, and players have to be trained to do that. Strict refereeing of the ruck and maul is important because collapse of the mauls can have serious consequences. The short arm tackle/high tackle has to be banned more forcibly. Foul play must be punished very harshly especially in international players who are setting the example. Running with the ball in both hands and using the head as a battering ram should be discouraged.

Discussion

GRAYSON: The medical matter fascinates me, bearing in mind we were talking about spinal injury with rotation. Can I enquire, is there any cross-fertilisation with your problems and all the work done by Gutman and his team at Stoke Mandeville for the last 45 year, because quite clearly, before 1940 there was no rehabilitation unit for spinal injuries as there is now because on the psychological factor, Gutman's philosophy has been very simple. The rehabilitation of bodies through the mind and participating in sports, you've now got the British Disability Sports Association and so forth. So my question is: is there any cross-fertilisation in trying to see how they have developed with their own broken bodies, for benefiting your more stable areas?

MOLLOY: Yes, there tends to be cross-fertilisation. There is discussion in most conferences dealing with neck problems. One would always have rehabilitation in dealing with neck problems. The Stoke Mandeville group are the people that have the most experience. There are units in Australia and New Zealand as well with a lot of experience and they do make recommendations and have very strong views about rugby. Many of them feel that rugby should be banned—it's a dangerous game, and shouldn't be allowed. All very strong views, and obviously more communication is important.

QUESTIONER: With the view that there's no place for steroids, should we also not say that there's no place for giving local anaesthetics before one is going to perform?

MOLLOY: I can give you my comment on that. I would not use local anaesthetic or steroids before competition. I do not think it helps anybody. Lots of players insist on it—they ask for it, but I personally would not give it. I think they should not play if they need something like that.

WALKDEN: It was forbidden from 1974. The resolution of the international board said if they can't play without that then they should not play.

O'BRIEN: Well, if you are going to have dope in control of the World Cup, you cannot give steroids and you cannot give local anaesthetics, if you are using the IOC rules. If you do give any type of injection, you must give a written submission and you've got to justify giving it. There are very few cases where you can justify it, and I think it's absolutely crazy. Even giving a homeopathic is wrong because the person believes you're giving something.

HUGO: Involving your front rankers to try and get through to the other players through the coaching people—it's not very easy because very often the coach thinks he is discrediting himself by bringing in an ex-player to try and talk to his players, so I think it's wrong and I think the coaches also need education.

MOLLOY: Yes, they do, and I feel like others here that if the coaches are involved in cardiopulmonary resuscitation, it will make them more aware of potential trouble, and perhaps make them a little more responsible. I'm not suggesting they are not but, make them think more carefully about it. We have already mentioned one of our players who was injured but the great tendency is to jump for the ball in the air. What are your views on that? How would you advise a young full-back, because there tend to be a lot of injuries from that, at all levels of rugby—they tend to jump and collect the ball when they are about to be taken by some on-rushing players.

WILLIAMS: Well, you're very susceptible and the *par excellence* is Australian Rules, where they are off the ground all of the time to take the ball. I think

[37]

you've just got to encourage players to keep their eyes on the ball but if the opponents are coming for your legs, then that can cause a lot of nasty injuries. This is where the referees have got to be very strict on people taking you out before the ball. I think that's a sending-off offence.

BURRY: That is an extremely good point. In fact, in Victoria, in Australian Rules, the incidence of serious cervical injury is extremely low, and I think you may have actually put your finger on the reason, that is that they really do not go for the legs because they are not allowed to tackle anybody below the waist. So, anybody who is going in, is supposed to go for the ball. They are allowed to obstruct other people going for the ball within reach and within a few feet but they can only go for top body contact.

McLATCHIE: You remarked on the importance of cardiopulmonary resuscitation and on the importance of updating skills at doing CPR. Studies done on both sides of the Atlantic show the more senior you become medically, the less competent you are at CPR, and the more likely you are to think that you are able to do it. I'd like to just emphasise the fact that we really need to update our core skills all the time, all of us. In fact, the studies that we've done in the United Kingdom showed that the most successful people at CPR were the housemen and the junior staff nurse on the ward, and that was ratified on the other side of the Atlantic where the more senior you become, the more cocky you become about doing it and the less competent. So, it's vital, I think that referees learn these skills and so should the doctor at the touch-line.

And the other point was really just a point of general interest. In 1978 we were interested in the development of osteoarthritis in joint loading. And we looked at former international weight-lifters who load their non-weight bearing joints. It was a very simple study, based on symptomatology with a control group for comparison and we looked for radiological changes.

Our findings were that these weight-lifters were at no greater risk of osteoarthritis than the population in general. In real terms they had less osteoarthritis than the others. What we did find was that—and it's in keeping with most other things—a previously injured joint is much more susceptible to osteoarthritis after heavy loading, but the sport itself did not seem to increase the risk of osteoarthritis.

HUGO: One thing that we should remember, 5 per cent of shoulder dislocations do have neurological problems, especially around the neck of the humerus. We saw two this season. Most of these recover. It is a very depressing injury for a young man to get his deltoid paralysed.

What I really wanted to talk about is the lumbar spine. Having seen a young player with spondylolisthesis, who had been playing rugby for the last few years with some discomfort in his low back: what would you do? Would you suggest that he go back to the game?

MOLLOY: A percentage of players at international level have this problem and manage very well.

HUGO: This sort of thing illustrates that you must treat the player and not just the X-ray. You show the X-ray to your orthopaedic colleagues and they say: 'He can no longer play', when he has been playing international rugby for years. It becomes more complicated if the player has a fusion of the spine. The consensus would be that we evaluate the approach individually.

ENGLAND: The catch with these X-rays is not that the problem is at the L5–S1 level. You have to look at what is happening at the disc space above. A player may have disc resorption and magnetic resonance imaging (MRI) would be useful in eliciting this. Then you have got to decide whether this is your problem.

CHASE: I went to a meeting on this at the American Spine Association and there was a prolonged discussion about whether student athletes could continue to play football. The consensus was no, they cannot, because of the rules which have already been set up. In general there was a lot of discussion about whether this was a source of their back pain or whether it was just an X-ray claim. They needed to follow serial films to see if the vertebrae are moving. If they are moving, they need to be fused. The main problem is whether it really is the source of back pain. In the US they are not allowed to play grid iron football with that injury.

HUGO: That is the law? A player may undergo discectomy and partial laminectomy. He is symptom-free, he has been off for the season and he wants to go back to play. What do you do? Do you say it is OK?

O'BRIEN: I do not think I would. It depends on the position that he is playing and whether he has any residual symptoms and good abdominal muscles.

WALKDEN: I think that you must have intensive physiotherapy to carry the injury along and review him again in about a year.

ENGLAND: I think that MRI using a stir sequence may help. A sequence which outlines the cerebrospinal fluid with a high intensity signal, may show no anterior indentation of the column. I also think that you need CT scan to be sure that there is no abnormality of the foraminal outlets.

HUGO: We are talking a lot about the nuclear magnetic techniques. I am fortunate to have a radiologist who is really interested only in the CT scan. We have been satisfied with the results on the lumbar spine. Let us look at the cervical spine. Just to remind us we are really looking at the spinal column—there are ligaments, the cord and structures outside the cord. To say something about the exercises. Do they do anything to the shoulder or to the cervical spine? It is said that in normal circumstances the forces on the cervical spine are dissipated by the energy capabilities of the muscles, the discs and to a lesser extent the ligaments.

When a force applied to the cervical spine exceeds the elastic capabilities of the involved structures, injuries occur. This is where the dissipation comes in. Mechanical injuries seem to be similar in most of the sports and we thought in rugby it was mostly the flexion and to a certain extent extension injury. In fact vertical compression causes column buckling. We do think that the strengthening of, or conditioning of, the muscles have a beneficial effect on prevention. We do not think that muscle build-up would compensate for a total tear.

What do we do for the cervical spine as a general practitioner? After examining the patient on the field—and we support the feeling that we should not try and rotate him or twist his neck on the field, we should take him off the way he is lying—one of the most important things is to get a proper X-ray. You have to obtain a full view to T1 level to see that all the vertebrae are level, because a low dislocation/subluxation can be missed. If you look at the X-rays you might say there is something wrong. It is not always easy. If you are worried about it you can do the other tests. I have always found that unless you are a radiologist you have difficulties. It is more important to appreciate displacement. In spite of good X-ray showing no deficit patients can still sublux in the subsequent period.

Following an injury to the cervical spine with a fracture or a dislocation a patient may have fusion. He wants to go back to the game. Do you let him play?

MOLLOY: No.

McLATCHIE: I agree. I would suggest that he shouldn't play.

CHASE: Where I come from, absolutely not! There are players who have gone back after anterior cervical interdiscal fusions. If you think a player has absolutely informed consent and is aware of all the alternatives—if you have a stable spine that you can prove on flexion-extension feels no symptoms, I think they probably would be allowed to go back.

DAVIES: Where would you stand legally if you have allowed this man to go back into a collision sport?

CHASE: Well, there are players who have gone back to grid iron with neck fusions. They have to appreciate that the incidence and chances of re-injury are greater than in a normal person.

HUGO: But, if a patient has been warned by the governing body that he is more prone to injury, and in spite of medical recommendation he prefers to play the game, does he by signing a form disassociate himself from the medical recommendation?

GRAYSON: In other words he exonerates the medical profession and the governing body. When I mentioned this at the Football Association conference, Bert Millerchip, the FA Chairman and a retired solicitor said: 'The best advice I ever gave was to say that if a doctor was going to warn a patient and/or the club about the risk of a potential player getting an injury, it is to put it in writing and the patient signs it, that is the best advice I could ever give'. The opportunity given to the player of knowing by informed consent what the consequences are, and a player notwithstanding that goes on, he is doing that at his own risk. He has got to be warned, but is taking the risk upon himself.

WALKDEN: I think that the last point is important. Full information should be given to the player because we have had two situations where the front row, one with calcification from a haemorrhage in the lower posterior ligament and another with a fracture, and one both felt without the consensus that you shouldn't really play them. You have to give the full explanation to the man, and to the selectors.

It has always seemed to me that in the thoracic and the lumbar spine, if you have got fusion of two vertebrae then there is scope for compensatory movement. I don't know whether it is a misconception or not, but it seems to me that a small alteration or restriction in the movement of the cervical spine has much greater biomechanical consequences. If you allow somebody to go back to the sort of rugby activity that in the future may be coupled with cervical vertebrae then you are putting them at greater risk of injuries above and below.

HUGO: A player with an incidental congenital fusion would be handled in the same way.

CHASE: I think you can point out to him that the disc above the fusion is at risk of breaking down.

HUGO: What about other neck injuries? A player falling onto his head with an anterior disc prolapse that we do not really recognise in rugby, but which has been well recognised in the American game. These include aspects of the 'burning hand syndrome' affecting the forearms as well. The peripheral nerves may be injured and simulate cervical spine problems. We very often find that these players are being examined, their cervical spine is being X-rayed and the doctors say afterward that a neck is so bad that the patient cannot play. We have to remind ourselves that these conditions are different and tend to improve. We have gone through a survey of 20 000 schoolboys in South Africa indicating that

[41]

almost half of them are not fit, and that thousands of schoolboys playing rugby should not be on the playing field. I think that the question of examining the player and scrutinising these individuals for possible injuries is very important.

It is important to undertake conventional discussion and comb the problems out, but I think that we should also expand the problem areas.

7: Head Injuries due to Sport and their Relevance to Rugby

G.R.McLATCHIE

THIS CHAPTER relates to work carried out over the past 12 years, initially in Glasgow and subsequently in the north of England. Head injuries may be categorised as serious (those requiring neurosurgical care), or 'trivial' (apparently not serious because the patient may appear to be normal), i.e. related to the extent of brain damage sustained which may be diffuse or focal. Primary brain damage results at the time of trauma and is irreversible. Secondary brain damage such as hypoxia, brain swelling, bleeding and infection may complicate the situation and lead to the death of the individual. These secondary changes may be reversible and are the reason for accurate observation of head-injured patients.

There are many situations in which head injuries can occur in sport. The injury may be accidental (i.e. not part of the rules of sport) as in soccer, football, hockey, horse riding, etc., or intentional either as part of the rules in boxing, or due to foul play, e.g. punching or kicking another player. Rugby is no exception to both accidental and intentional injury [1]. We should therefore anticipate that head injury may be a feature of rugby medicine and give warning to the various controlling bodies.

We reviewed the case notes of all patients with sports-related head injuries admitted to the Institute of Neurological Sciences in Glasgow from 1974 to 1978 [2]. This serves a population of 2.7 million people. Only 52 (2.7% of all admissions) were due to sport. The sports most frequently causing injury were golf, horse riding and football (Table 7.1). Only three were due to rugby and two patients made a good recovery. The high incidence of golf-related injuries can be explained when one considers the popularity of the sport in Scotland and the fact that the average age of the players was 10 years. The injuries were all depressed skull fractures and were sustained by the players standing too close to their colleagues who were wielding golf clubs.

Traditionally, we regard concussion as a minor injury which is reversible. However, we know from boxers that recurrent minor head injuries can be cumulative in effect and lead to the punch drunk syndrome well recognised in the thirties and forties in professional booth boxers [3]. Hawkeye Pearce (in the TV series *MASH*) said that he always wanted to keep his senility for his old age. Unfortunately many boxers develop it when they are still young.

A postal enquiry in the north of England showed that only a small number of rugby players with concussion or post-traumatic amnesia are admitted to hospital; of 303 players with head injuries, 58 had post-traumatic amnesia (PTA) for more than 1 hour and 232 for more than 5 minutes. Only 38 of these were admitted to hospital. Many continued to play after 'recovery'; some were unable to resume work for 3 or 4 weeks or said they did not cope well; some did not even want to play rugby again. This so-called post-traumatic syndrome may persist for several weeks after a minor head injury [4].

When young rugby players who had sustained minor head injuries were

Table 7.1 Frequency of head injury due to sport from a survey conducted in Glasgow over 5 years [2]. Figures in parentheses show results as a percentage of total number of cases

Sport	No. of cases	Good	Moderately disabled	Severely disabled	Died
Golf	14	14 (100)	—	—	—
Horse-riding	8	5 (63)	2 (25)	1 (13)	—
Football	7	6 (86)	1 (14)	—	—
Shooting	5	5 (100)	—	—	—
Climbing	4	3 (75)	—	—	1 (25)
Rugby	3	2 (67)	1 (32)	—	—
Boxing	2	2 (100)	—	—	—
Skating	2	2 (100)	—	—	—
Others	7	6 (86)	—	1 (14)	—
Total	52	45 (86)	4 (8)	2 (4)	1 (2)

Table 7.2 The Glasgow Coma Scale as recommended by the author for assessment of rugby head injuries

Function	Response
Eye opening	Spontaneous
	To speech
	To pain
	None
Best verbal response	Orientated
	Confused conversation
	Inappropriate words
	Incomprehensible sounds
	None
Best motor response	Obeys commands
	Localizes
	Flexes
	Extends
	None

studied in New Zealand [5] it was noted that they had impaired psychological function for 2–3 weeks after injury and although they suffered only a few minutes PTA this may be related to traumatic microscopic structural brain damage [6]. Players reinjured within 2 or 3 weeks took longer to recover their mental acuity [7]. Is it possible, then, that recurrent minor head injuries in sports other than boxing could lead to a syndrome similar to traumatic encephalopathy? It appears that those cells damaged do not recover but others take over their function. It then becomes a matter of arithmetic. The more head injuries, the more neuronal damage. The effects are cumulative.

Our recommendations for combat and contact sports are firstly, prevent minor head injury itself, and secondly, prevent cumulative brain damage. Referees, coaches, trainers and players must be aware of the implications of minor head injuries. We therefore made a recommendation that there should be a 4 week lay-off after a minor head injury to allow psychological recovery. One solution in rugby would be to encourage the use of substitutes at all levels; encourage the concept of a first team pool rather than just a first team. If there is neurological impairment which is measurable then a patient should not return to his former sport until such times as he has been seen and examined by a specialist in neurological or neurosurgery. If there has been a severe head injury there should be no return to that contact or combat sport.

Assessment of head injuries

How do you assess head injuries? The method that we use and recommend is the Glasgow Coma Scale [8]. It has now been accepted world-wide as a measure of neurological function (Table 7.2). There are three parameters; (a) what the patient's eyes do; (b) what the patient's best motor response is; and (c) whether or not he talks sense.

Prevention of brain damage

How do you prevent brain damage? If a patient has PTA or has been knocked out then some form of brain damage has occurred and the patient should be seen in the accident and emergency (A & E) department where a skull radiograph should be performed. If a fracture is present, admission is recommended because of a slightly increased risk of sustaining an intracranial haemorrhage.

What other methods can you use? Head gear in boxing prevents knock-out and possibly reduces the risk of intracranial bleeding [9]. Paradoxically, because it protects against knock-out, it may increase the risk of recurrent head injury. The rules of boxing prohibit fighting for the rest of a year if there is a history of three knock-outs but if a fighter is never knocked out he may sustain multiple PTAs with no apparent ill effect. Head gear is good for preventing cuts about the eye but may be of no value at all in preventing encephalopathy.

American studies looked at various aspects of sporting helmet design [10,11]. Steeple-chase jockeys may develop encephalopathy after frequent falls [12,13]. The Jockey Club changed the rules and they now wear the mini motorcycle crash helmets that jockeys wear. When that helmet was adopted as a British standard for girls doing social riding their head injury incidence was also reduced. Thus, changing the rules of the sport and the type of safety gear can change the incidence of head injury.

In 1974, a questionnaire was sent to 165 British neurologists asking whether any had ever seen a condition that looks like the punch drunk syndrome in any sportsmen? Boxing was incriminated again but neurologists felt that soccer players would repay systematic enquiry [3]. The professional soccer player may head the ball up to 2000 times in a season. Swedish work has suggested that professional soccer players may be at high risk of traumatic encephalopathy (unpublished).

In view of the regular denials that amateur boxers are immune to brain damage we decided to examine a small group [14]. Examinations were done by a consultant neurologist at the Institute of Neurology. Electroencephalographic (EEG) examination, computerised tomographic (CT) scanning and neuropsychometric techniques were employed. Twenty boxers with an average age of 25 volunteered for the study. Clinical examination was abnormal in 35%; the EEG was abnormal in 40%, CT scan was abnormal in only one out of 20. Neuropsychometry in 16 who underwent these mental acuity tests detected abnormality in 50%. The EEG abnormality was twice that which would be expected in normal people and neuropsychometry was radically different from controls. One interpretation is that people who take up boxing already have brain damage. Most derive from social classes 4 and 5 and have fought all their lives. It could also mean that brain damage is caused by boxing. We found a significant correlation between brain dysfunction and the number of fights; under 40 fights, there seemed to be fewer abnormalities.

We would thus advocate that the best methods for evaluating head injury are clinical examination using the Glasgow Coma Scale for acute trauma, and neuropsychological testing for detecting significant degrees of brain damage in sportsmen.

Discussion

CHASE: First of all in boxing, but also in rugby, there is something called second impact syndrome. I wonder if this is the post-traumatic syndrome which you were talking about?

McLATCHIE: If you do sustain a minor head injury, you are much more likely to sustain a second one and that was one of the reasons why the player really should be taken off the park. Certainly if he took part in rugby during the 4 week recovery period again he is likely to be more injury prone. Head injury leads itself to further injury and recurrent problems.

CHASE: In the second impact syndrome, as I understood it, the patient has suffered a head injury and then a subsequent injury can be catastrophic. An example was a boy who stopped playing rugby for 3 weeks and I wonder if we should extend that.

McLATCHIE: I think probably 3 weeks is reasonable. Unlike boxing, rugby is not a sport in which head injury is the intention. We have made recommendations for various sports. In karate it is 4 months which means that a player after a minor head injury is out for the rest of the season.

GILFEATHER: For the Rugby Union it is a minimum of 21 days after which there is a neurological examination by a doctor.

CHASE: What type of examination is that and how much psychometric testing? Is there a standardised test for clearance?

McLATCHIE: I think there is no psychometric testing.

WALKDEN: The medical advisory committee of the International Rugby

Board recommended, and this is what is printed, that a return to rugby requires a minimum of 3 weeks and then only after a full neurological examination has been carried out. A neurological examination can be carried out by a medical practitioner—it does not imply a neurologist. The implication is that there is something in the laws of the game that head injury precludes playing, but that is not correct. There is only a recommendation.

WALKDEN: It's a resolution. The Medical Advisory Committee of the International Rugby Board strenuously encouraged the IRB to change the laws of the game to preclude people from playing; a mandatory stand-down period for 3 weeks. They declined and so at the moment there is a recommendation.

MCLATCHIE: This is why it's so important that referees know the implications of minor head injuries.

CHASE: There are two important points: (1) we don't have a law that makes it mandatory, and (2) we don't have a standardised form of examination.

MCLATCHIE: The other comment I'd like to make to you about psycho-metric testing is that it has now progressed so that a rapid card system of basic tests can be used. These test recall, processing of information and regurgitation of information at various levels. It can be matched for age, intellect and social class and it's reproducible.

O'BRIEN: We found that CT scans in boxers can be normal, but antibodies to brain may be raised after competition when CT scans are normal.

CHASE: Would MRI be of more value?

O'BRIEN The problem with the MRI is that it costs £500 000 and people haven't got the money.

GRAYSON: These are several points which Greg created (we will pick them up in my own address). There are a number of interesting ones which I need to briefly discuss in the meantime. Greg has touched upon a crucial thing which is very rarely understood in the sporting administration because they don't use their brains when they administer sport because they don't in their usual businesses. That is, the fundamental difference between the playing laws of the game and in the administrative laws and the penal playing laws, and the interesting point you make which is relevant to not only head injuries but other injuries, is having a group so a substitute can come on and prevent an ordinary knock upon any part of the anatomy being exacerbated by having to go on playing. That to my mind, is a crucial point which shows the differential between playing laws and the administrative laws. Which goes on to the mandatory direction for medical examination, which again in an administrative law particularly for the penal playing law, and the correlating point is of course that we can talk about educating the referees. But then of course, you've got to educate not only the referee, but also the coaches and the team groups for the lower level of the game rather than the public level of what you might call 'social rugby'.

Someone mentioned insurance. Well, it is very interesting that one of the most progressive moves for school rugby at a young level, came as a result of the very important recommendation of MOSA (the Medical Officers Schools Association) in 1978, which gave rise to the direction that all schools should be insured against rugby injuries. That gave rise to a very interesting piece of education I'll mention. About that time the British Medical Association came up with the recommendation for the abolition of boxing, because there was a great conflict in the medical world. The Public Schools' Medical Association also recommended the abolition of boxing and as I understand it, with the retirement of the coach at Clifton School, no public school now indulges in boxing. I think that Oxford and Cambridge still have a boxing competition, but the question I would like to put to you is this; do you go as far as the British Medical Association in the recommendation of banning boxing, or do you have a sort of qualification of it because of not withstanding injuries?

McLATCHIE: There is no doubt at all that boxing produces brain damage, but you really have to make quality decisions about this. For instance, is it better for a social class 4 or 5 boy to have the discipline of boxing (which is what the coach in training argues) and sustain the very small risk of death in the ring, against the risk of getting lung cancer or heart disease in his early forties? We also did a corollary to the boxing study. We looked at smoking habits of social class 4 and 5 people, and only 1.7% of boxers were smokers against a predicted percentage of 42%. What we do not know is whether after he stopped boxing he reverted to the norm of his peer group. There may be an ethical question about doctors being involved in boxing, and it may be comparable to doctors being involved in torture. Almost by definition, doctors should stop a fight as soon as the first punch is landed. I just wonder whether or not doctors who are now involved in boxing are, in fact, acting ethically? The other thing that I would suggest is that if doctors are not involved in boxing, it would not as everyone says go underground—it would collapse and die, because there would be no more multi-million pound fights; there would be no media world championship fights. How do you keep a multi-million pound fight underground? I think that if doctors were not associated with boxing it would not be so popular as it is today.

BATH UNIVERSITY MEDICAL OFFICER: I have an observation really. As a medical officer to the University at Bath, I have attempted to get boxing eliminated from the sporting programme at that university, bringing forward a lot of the arguments that Greg cited. The question I would like to ask is what does recovery imply? This 3-week interval at the end of which there is a normal neurological examination; does that mean that they are then less likely to suffer the cumulative effects of further head injuries?

McLATCHIE: Not really. All that we know is that there has probably been anatomical damage, and the remaining brain cells have taken over. It takes about 3 or 4 weeks for that function to return. To you and me these people look normal and they act normally. I would suggest that if they continue to box, brain damage will have become significant after about 40 bouts. We have used the term 'brain damage' too often. I think we have got to quantify. This is what people want to know—when does it matter? For instance, Jim Watt, the World Professional Light-weight Champion said that he may well be brain damaged but he does not wake up in the morning and use his toothbrush to clean his forehead! He was a bright boxer, and the answer was that Jim Watt probably started off with a lot more brain cells than many boxers and he's lost some of them. It doesn't matter—he's still a man of high intellect. If he had continued in boxing he would have become 'punch drunk'.

CHASE: That brings up the interesting question of maybe only the smartest people should box!

References

1 Davies JE, Gibson T. Injuries in rugby union football. *Br Med J* 1978; **ii:** 1759.
2 Lindsay KW, McLatchie GR, Jennett B. Serious head injury in sport. *Br Med J* 1980; **281:** 789.
3 Corsellis JAN. Brain damage in sport. *Lancet* 1974; **i:** 401.
4 Cook JB. The effects of minor head injuries sustained in sport and the postconcussional syndrome. In: Walker AE, Caverness WF, Critchley M, eds. *The Late Effects of Head Injury*. Illinois: CC Thomas, 1969: 408.
5 Gronwall D, Wrightson P. Delayed recovery of intellectual function after minor head injury. *Lancet* 1974; **ii:** 605.
6 Oppenheimer DR. Microscopic lesions in the brain following head injury. *J Neurol Neurosurg Psych* 1968; **31:** 299.
7 Gronwall D, Wrightson P. Cumulative effect of concussion. *Lancet* 1975; **ii:** 995.
8 Teasdale G, Jennett B. Assessment of coma and impaired consciousness: a practical scale. *Lancet* 1974; **ii:** 81.
9 Schmid L, Hajiik E, Votipka F, Teprik O, Bloustein JL. Experience with headgear in boxing. *J Sports Med Phys Fitness* 1968; **8:** 171.
10 Clark K, Powell J. Football helmets and neurotrauma—an epidemiological overview of three seasons. *Med Sci Sports* 1979; **11:** 138.

11 Dooley BJ, Trinca GW. Value of protective headgear in reducing head injuries. In: Heulke DF, ed. *Proc Am Assoc Automot Med* 22nd Conference, Illinois: AAAM, 1978: 49.

12 Foster JB, Leiguarda R, Tilley PJB. Brain damage in national hunt jockeys. *Lancet* 1976; **i**: 981.

13 Allen W. Brain damage in jockeys. *Lancet* 1976; **i**: 1135.

14 McLatchie GR, Brooks N, Galbraith S *et al.* Clinical neurological examination, neuropsychology, electro-encephalography and computed tomographic head scanning in active amateur boxers. *J Neurol Neurosurg Psych* 1987; **50**: 96.

8: Studies of Concussion and Equilibrium function

I. KONO

INJURIES can be anticipated in rugby football because of the nature of the game and concussion is a matter of concern. The note in Law 3 states that a player who has suffered definite concussion should not participate in any match or training for a period of at least 3 weeks from the time of injury and then only subject to being cleared by proper neurological examination. Concussion is a clinical syndrome characterised by immediate impairment of neurological functions such as consciousness, vision, motion and sensation [1].

There is a spectrum of concussion from mild to severe. In Japan, rugby football is rapidly growing in popularity. Today there are 120 000 players. An initial survey of concussion was undertaken in 2000 players during the season 1987–88. Approximately 20% of the players suffered concussion, an extraordinarily large number. Tackles accounted for 60% and being tackled accounted for 16%. Only 40% of players left the field. About half of the players concussed suffered some persistent symptoms. About 20% suffered longer than 3 weeks, and about 26% less than 3 weeks. In this survey, loss of consciousness occurred in 47% of players, post-traumatic amnesia or retrograde amnesia in 70%, and headaches or unsteadiness in 70%. Unsteadiness includes subjective symptoms. In view of the frequency of unsteadiness, functional test for body balance (equilibrium function) was undertaken in 39 players—17 without and 22 with a concussion history, over 4 years. Controls were 29 students of the University of Tsukaba, School of Physical Education, 12 of whom were gymnasts.

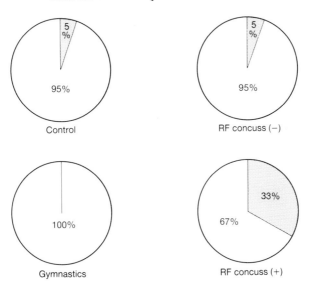

Fig. 8.1 Mann test. RF concuss (+)/(−)=rugby players with/without a history of concussion. (▨) Poor, (□) normal.

The Mann test, the one foot long-standing test, the stepping test and the tandem gait test were used. The Mann test involves standing in a heal-to-toe position with the dominant behind the non-dominant foot, with eyes open or closed. If the subject moved his feet from the given position or opened his eyes on the 'eyes closed' phase before reaching the maximum balance time of 30 seconds the test was positive. Amongst the controls, 5% showed poor function, and all who were gymnasts performed the test perfectly (Fig. 8.1). Of the rugby football players without concussion, 5% had poor test results. However, 33% of those with a history of concussion had poor function. The average time for standing was 15 seconds.

The one foot standing test involves standing on the right foot with eyes open or with eyes closed. The test was concluded if the foot moved or touched the suspended foot on the ground, if the suspended foot was used for support, if the subject opened his eyes on the 'eyes closed' trial, or if the subject reached the maximum balance time of 30 seconds. Amongst the controls about 30% showed poor results, but 100% of the gymnasts performed perfectly. Of the rugby players without concussion, 27% were abnormal (Fig. 8.2). About half of the concussed players showed poor function tests.

In rugby football, there are many occasions such as in jumping and kicking the ball when well controlled body balance is essential for safety and for keeping the ball. The stressed one foot standing test involves standing on

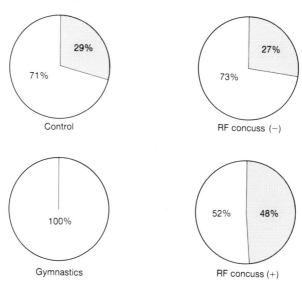

Fig. 8.2 One foot standing test with eyes closed. RF concuss (+)/(−)=rugby players with/without a history of concussion. (▨) Poor, (□) normal.

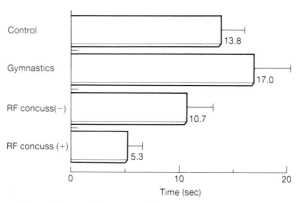

Fig. 8.3 Stressed one foot standing test with eyes closed after jumping with rotation. Values expressed as mean±SE. RF concuss (+)/(−)=rugby players with/without a history of concussion.

one leg just after jumping with rotation as in a line-out. Players with a history of concussion could not stand for longer than 5 seconds on average (Fig. 8.3). Gymnastic students could stand on average for 17 seconds.

In the stepping test, subjects stepped 100 times on a mark with eyes closed. The distance moved from the mark is normally less than 1 m. Again, half of the players with a history of concussion showed a poorer result.

In the tandem gait test, subjects walk along a line with eyes closed.

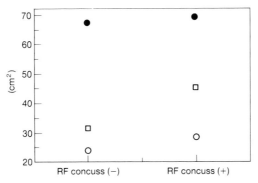

Fig. 8.4 Area included within the sway path of the central pressure. Values are mean area for a period of 25 seconds keeping Mann posture (□), one foot standing with eyes open (○) and closed (●). RF concuss (+)/(−)=rugby players with/without a history of concussion.

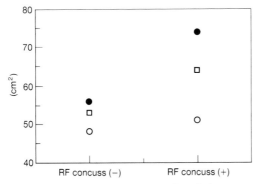

Fig. 8.5 Length of the head sway. Values are mean length for a period of 25 seconds keeping Mann posture (□), one foot standing with eyes open (○) and closed (●). RF concuss (+)/(−)=rugby players with/without a history of concussion.

Normal deflection from the line must not exceed 1 m. Players with a history of concussion deflected a greater distance than the others.

From the results of these function tests, rugby football players with a history of concussion appeared to have defective equilibrium function. To confirm the results of the clinical function tests, stability tests were performed on a force platform, with the collaboration of Professor Asami of the University of Tsukuba, Institute of Health and Sport Sciences. This tested swaying of the body and head. The momentum of force generated by the ankle muscle to keep the body in the right position is equal to central pressure as measured through a force platform plate [2, 3]. The length of the sway path and the area included in the sway path were studied. Sampling time was 50 milliseconds. Sway of the head measurement utilised a mobile bar. Sampling time was 50 milliseconds. A software program was designed to analyse these data on microcomputer. The mobile bar was attached to the head and connected to a sensor so that when the subject swayed, the mobile recorded the length and direction of sway. The false plate on which the subject stood recorded the pressure distribution.

Subjects were five players without and eight players with a history of concussion within the previous 2 years. The area included within the sway path of central pressure was wider in players with a history of concussion than in players without concussion (Fig. 8.4). The head swayed greater in players with a history of concussion than in players without concussion (Fig. 8.5). These results showed that rugby players with a history of concussion showed poor results in stability tests.

Functional tests were performed prospectively in 70 players at the beginning of the season in 1989–90. There were four players concussed in this season. One sustained concussion in tackling; loss of consciousness was 1–2 minutes with no further loss of memory. Computerised tomography (CT) scan was normal. The Mann test on the day of concussion was 36 seconds, but returned to normal the next day. However, the one foot standing test took 1 week to return to normal. In the second case a 20-year-old winger with no previous history of concussion, sustained 6 minutes loss of consciousness in a tackle. In this case, stressed one foot standing test was abnormal for an extended period. The third case had a history of concussion and the current episode was also sustained in tackling. There was no loss of consciousness, but a slight retrograde amnesia. The CT scan was normal. Function tests were abnormal. The fourth player was a 21-year-old scrum-half. He had a history of concussion, often in tackling with loss of consciousness for 2–3 minutes and loss of memory. He had a normal CT scan. In this case there was a delay in returning to normal for every parameter.

From these results it is apparent that concussion does have an effect on equilibrium function for a period in rugby football players. Further investigation is required to determine whether these effects are cumulative. It is essential for the referee to apply strictly the guidelines especially in younger players and the medical profession must advise on a return to the field [4].

Discussion

CHASE: This brings up important information. It is very unnerving to think that 60% of the players who have suffered a concussion did not leave the field. That has been my own experience and I think that we must do something to improve that statistic at all levels of rugby. Forty-five per cent of those players who did not leave the field were symptomatic some weeks after the incident, which we've already heard puts them at great risk from additional injury. The 30% of those that were studied and were abnormal with a history of concussion—I'd like to ask how long after the concussion were they studied?

It was also clear here that unconsciousness is not necessarily the indication of a head injury. We should probably expand how we evaluate the player who has had a head injury.

I noticed that statistics presented here indicate that there were symptoms and findings in concussed players at least up to 2 years later. When should these players return and how should they be tested? How dangerous is the tackle? Perhaps gymnasts should be those who are encouraged to play rugby. The more sensitive the tests, the more abnormalities are picked up and for a longer time.

O'BRIEN: Did any of those people who stood on one leg have ankle injuries prior to that, because if you've had an ankle injury that is not treated properly you would get the same type of result.

KONO: Some of the players suffered ankle injuries but these showed good results.

BURRY: When you do the Mann test and the one foot standing test, do you give them a practice at it first and do they have a time to get used to doing the test?

KONO: Yes, some of these tests can be used for rehabilitation of poor body balance.

ETIENNE: You didn't answer John Chases's question about the timing of the test in relation to the concussion. How long after a concussion episode were these tests performed?

KONO: It is an important point. Some of the players were concussed years ago.

ETIENNE: It is therefore possible, that concussion might result in permanent dysfunction.

KONO: Yes I think so. Further investigation is necessary.

CHASE: Does the immediate treatment of head injury influence results later?

McLATCHIE: I really don't know that. The standard approach has always been that patients should be in bed resting for, say 24 hours. Certainly, those who go to hospital with suspected skull fractures are kept in for, say 24 hours on bed rest. Whether that makes any difference to your brain at the end of the day, I just don't know.

WALKDEN: I think we can recommend some amendment to Law 3. The alteration of the words 'should not participate' should be 'must not participate', and secondly we should work out and devise psychometric testing and equilibrium testing and present these as firm recommendations. Does the duration of amnesia relate to the management of the concussed case?

KONO: I can't find any relation.

DAVIES: I know that you are concerned about head injury rates in Japan. There are few pitches for 120 000 players and in the summer these grounds are very hard. Could you tell us about your Kanto Medical Society?

KONO: Rugby is very popular in Japan so, to cope with this situation, we established the Kanto Medical Society in 1982. The society comprises about 200 rugby doctors. The aims of the society are:

1 To deliver doctors to the field and in the Kanto area, we serve every game around the city;

2 To handle the statistics;

3 To arrange emergency systems in this area; and

4 To handle academic aspects of rugby medicine. We act completely as a voluntary group and so we have many organisational problems. We could provide some of the other unions with suggestions.

ENGLAND: In the RFU, there is a mandatory requirement for a player after a concussion to rest from his sport for 21 days. Should we consider 28 days to be more appropriate or is 21 realistic?

McLATCHIE: Boxers have always had 4 weeks off and by chance, it seems to take that long to recover psychometric function. Our contention in rugby football that 3 weeks is satisfactory was based on the fact that rugby football is not a sport in which head injury is the end point. I did say also that, in karate, they over-reacted and laid them off for months. I think it's probably worthwhile rethinking; there must be more work done now on psychometric testing after minor head injuries and it may well be that a 4-week period would be satisfactory.

WALKDEN: I just want to clarify a fact. Is there any rugby union throughout the world, where it is mandatory for 3 weeks to be off so is it still, *should* be or *must* be?

McLATCHIE: I think this is very important. We really have to decide how we act as a body—whether we are authoritarian or whether we are advising.

CHASE: In the case of head injury, I don't think there's any question ethically.

GRAYSON: Absolutely. I was fascinated by Dr Walkden's comments about the mandatory, as distinct from the discretionary factor, because in the professional game you have not the restraint to change regulations. These are defensible on the basis that it is reasonable for the protection of an organisation such as a sport and there is no doubt at all that if medical opinion and medical evidence establish that it is inherently dangerous for the participants to go back on the field after a certain injury, it will be in the interest of the community and the patient to make disqualification mandatory for those who are unfit to participate. There is no doubt at all that the law will support you.

BURRY: That's very encouraging because it was argued when we put the subject to the IRFB that it wouldn't stand up legally. If that is not so we would need to have stringent criteria for deciding that a player could be specifically prohibited from participating.

GRAYSON: I think you'd have to work out the definition.

References

1 Gennarelli TA. Cerebral concussion and diffuse brain injuries. In: Cooper PR, ed. *Head Injury*. Baltimore: Williams & Wilkins, 1987: 108–24.
2 Ekdahl C, Jarnolo GB, Andersson SI. Standing balance in healthy subjects. *Scand J Rehab Med* 1989; **21:** 187–95.
3 Winter DA, Patla AE, Frank JS. Assessment of balance control in humans. *Med Prog Technol* 1990; **16:** 31–51.
4 Cantu RC. Guidelines for return to contact sports after a cerebral concussion. *Physic Sports Med* 1986; **14:** 221–8.

9: Shoulder Injuries in Rugby

PATRICK ENGLAND

SHOULDER lesions account for 9–13% of all rugby injuries. An appreciation of the anatomy and range of movement is important to the diagnosis and management of shoulder problems. Adequate X-ray facilities are essential. Plain radiography should include the whole region so that low fractures or subluxations are not overlooked. Arthrographs may illustrate tears of the rotator cuff. Scans may be helpful. Ultrasonography is used but it has some disadvantages in that although it is non-invasive, it is still relatively imprecise. The three planes of magnetic resonance imaging (MRI) do provide excellent information, particularly of the rotator cuff and labrum. It will allow recognition of joint effusions and other damage to the soft tissue.

The vast majority of shoulder injuries are represented by contusion or bruising and resolve rapidly. Some do not; lesions of the acromioclavicular (AC) joint are seen particularly in the ball carrier rather than the tackler. He is often tackled, brought down and pinioned onto a shoulder. If the ball carrier tries to pass as he goes down, he is presenting the shoulder to the impact point and this accounts for many AC injuries. The pitch surface can also influence this injury. During the course of a tournament on an artificial surface, 33 injuries were recorded and a considerable number were to the AC joint. A lot of these injuries do not require intervention. There may be some permanent damage to the AC joint and some impingement of the capsule but many are asymptomatic and will subsequently take the impact of tackling and falling. The important joints, the ligaments, the conoid and trapezoid, remain intact and conservative management will suffice. When the conoid and trapezoid ligaments are disrupted and the shoulder drops, repair must be attempted or if recognised late the outer end of the clavicle can be excised. One way to determine whether this is significant or not is by putting a load-bearing weight onto the target shoulder and even with a small fragment broken off the lower end of the clavicle it will recover if the shoulder does not drop. Spacing may occur but the width of the AC joint is not important. However, where there is significant movement, operative reduction and fixation are required. It is then necessary to repair the ligaments and hold them simply for 4 weeks. When the outer end of the clavicle has been excised a reasonable shape can be achieved and even a forward can play again.

The supraspinatus tendon commonly tears about 1 centimetre proximal to the attachment in the tuberosity of the humerus and this is the critical area; there is upper subluxation of the head of the humerus which is diagnostic in late cases. In some shoulder injuries where there is persistent pain, in which there may be a painful arc which does not respond to the usual remedial therapy, one should think of what additional problem may exist. Is there perhaps some problem with the rotator cuff? It can occur in young individuals such as swimmers, gymnasts, props and racket players who over-use their shoulders. This may be termed a stage 1 lesion impingement.

Aching, a painful arc, a history of over-use, or a specific injury may be apparent and pathologically there is oedema and haemorrhage in the subacromial bursa which, if persistent will lead to fibrosis with thickening and a stage 2 lesion.

Stage 2 occurs commonly at about age 24 onwards. In older players, there may be difficulty with constant scrummaging and training, particularly if it involves a lot of weights. Chronic thickening of the subacromial bursa occurs and with time, wear of the rotator cuff. There may or may not be an obvious exostosis of the acromium in stage 2.

At age 40 or more there is further degeneration of the rotator cuff, leading to incomplete or full thickness tears, the stage 3 lesion. MRI views of lesions may reveal tears of the rotator cuff with evidence of fluid within the cuff itself, the tendon and the surrounding tissues. When arthrography is used, a computerised tomography (CT) scan should be incorporated but it may not identify a lesion deep to the acromial arc. MRI is therefore a better investigation.

In the early stage of the rotator cuff or impingement syndrome, physiotherapy and non-steroidal anti-inflammatories can be successful. Swollen debris and tissue can be cleared by an arthroscopic technique. Commonly it is necessary to divide the AC ligament in order to decompress the area.

In the later stages, where there is an exostosis, the same technique may be used with removal of the exostosis with a shaver and decompression of the coracoacromial ligament. In the third stage, where there are frank rotator cuff tears, an open procedure has to be employed although arthroscopy may be successful occasionally.

Dislocation is not as common as is often thought and management is conventional. Lesions may be difficult to identify even with techniques such as CT arthrography. A clue may be seen on rotational X-ray; the labrum may be torn from the glenoid and the head seen to be constantly subluxing. MRI images may reveal tears of the labrum. Posterior tears are not common and those of the sub-glenoid even less so.

Common fractures can be dealt with easily and require no surgery. Pinning may be necessary. A bony segment of the glenoid rim may be separated. It can be dealt with by screwing. Segmental, shattered fractures of the acromium can occur and are best dealt with by transfixion or plating.

Discussion

CHASE: What about the role of protective gear?

ENGLAND: Protective garments may be a hazard to anyone with whom the player collides. It is disadvantageous because it may encourage him to play when he is not fully fit. We have had, in informal discussion and formal discussion, examples of people who will hide injuries, so I think that any protective wear, from the waist upwards, is not a good thing. You will undoubtedly, if you do not think it is going to hurt you with a shoulder pad, or a harness, go in harder. You are going to do yourself more harm and you may well harm the other player. I would certainly not condone them. In practice or in training it may give you the opportunity of finding out whether a player is fit enough.

DAVIES: Do we have any evidence or any information from rugby league on shoulder injuries? As you know a lot of these players actually do wear protective padding.

ENGLAND: I can't answer that.

CHASE: I think it is very important, particularly in the shoulder that a full assessment and a documentation of the vascular status is done by the person who is going to perform the relocation. If you have not identified a neurological deficit in the arm—or a vascular one for that matter before you reduce it, and there is one after you reduce it, then you created it. Also, remember that axillary, suprascapular and long thoracic nerves do get injured in shoulder dislocations.

O'BRIEN: If players lift weights, with a lot of internal rotation and are not doing enough external rotation this may lead to posterior subluxation. If you get a pain around the shoulders, it is important to assess the external rotators to see whether there is a marked imbalance.

MACAIG: Fiji will never be able to afford an MRI, so, I think you can make a lot of these diagnoses clinically. In the chronic rotator cuff tears of those I have operated on, almost inevitably I have not been able to get the torn bits together again, so it is not as straightforward as it may seem. AC injuries are common but there is still no consensus of how one should treat them. Each year two or three articles are published, one for and one against operating. I am a non-operator and I think people have shown that long-term problems are cosmetic and very little else.

ENGLAND: Yes, that's a very fair point if I may answer that. First of all, I agree that not everybody can have the facility of MRI but I hope this may become available for most people. You can learn quite a lot with ultrasonography. This requires only a skilled operator; it is not really expensive so that is something that you could get organised to help you. With regard to acromioclavicular surgery, I agree, I am largely a waiter. I think it is really dependent on an individual's experience and as I have indicated, I think you can get better results by operating on some, and they do well.

CHASE: The two most important tests are external rotation and strength in the shoulder—they are almost all showing a weak external rotation at the cuff. The other thing is if the patient feels pain in the shoulder and you cannot determine the status of the rotator cuff I suggest that an injection of local anaesthetic will relieve pain and allow movement. If it doesn't then something is wrong.

ENGLAND: Yes, I think that would probably show a stage 2 where there is fibrosis occurring already because in stage 1 it wouldn't necessarily show that.

CHASE: The other thing that you mention which is also important is the thickening fibrosis. That can be a very difficult thing to treat.

ENGLAND: I would have no objection to a pad over an AC injury or even injection of the AC joint.

WALKDEN: If a player is recovering from injury at the AC joint he is permitted under law to apply a sponge rubber padding inside the little pocket on his shoulder.

ENGLAND: If you do this you must be sure that the player is not actually going to be putting himself at risk and is fit enough to play.

BURRY: There was a totally over-hysterical reaction to a photograph of a man with striking features connected to bones and screws which were even harder. He used to wear a harness across his shoulder, not to protect himself but to protect his opponents. When the photograph was taken he was actually leaning slightly forward and it looked as if his harness came right down over his skin, but it was actually the shadow of his shoulder pad. He was rather narrow across the shoulders.

PART 3
INVESTIGATION, TREATMENT AND OUTCOME

10: Athroscopic Knee Surgery and Ligament Replacement

J.P.R.WILLIAMS

I FIRST became interested in injuries to the knee when I sustained an injury myself in 1974. It transpired that I had torn my right posterior cruciate ligament and I declined surgery. Thankfully, I think it was the correct solution because I was able to play in the 1974 British Lions tour to South Africa without any problems.

The important structures are the menisci and the cruciate ligaments. On the lateral side there is a distance between the meniscus and the ligament. On the medial side they are in close proximity. The anterior cruciate ligament runs from the anterior tibial spine to the lateral femoral condyle and the posterior cruciate from the posterior tibial spine to the medial femoral condyle. The under surface of the patella is also important.

Lateral meniscal cysts to not always cause symptoms and are often an incidental finding. When I first started in orthopaedic surgery, symptomatic lateral meniscal cysts were treated by open total menisectomy. This is not done today. The mechanism of meniscal injury is flexion and rotation. It has been common in the mining fraternity and in sport. It is commoner in association football than in rugby football. The soccer players are more often on a flexed knee while rotating.

Three basic types of tear can occur. The peripheral detachment is particularly common on the medial side because of the close attachment of the medial ligament. The 'bucket-handle' tear or the 'bowstring' tear give rise to the classical symptom of a locked knee, i.e. inability to fully extend the joint. The tag tears occur in either the posterior, middle, or anterior part of the cartilage.

I was taught as a medical student that the menisci have no blood supply. That is true of the inner rim and explains why a synovial effusion occurs rather than bleeding into the joint. A peripheral detachment induces bleeding so it is not true that haemarthrosis cannot occur as a result of a cartilage tear. It has been known for some time that removing the whole of the meniscus leads to early 'wear and tear'. The meniscus was previously considered to be of no functional use. Perhaps one day we'll find that the appendix has some sort of usefulness! The history and clinical examination are important in meniscal injuries. Arthrography and arthroscopy are the standard investigations. I was fortunate to obtain a 6-month fellowship in sports medicine and knee surgery with Doug Jackson in Long Beach, California in 1981. He taught arthroscopic surgery without having the long learning curve of moving from diagnostic to operative arthroscopy. I find it difficult not to use a tourniquet. In Scandinavia a lot of arthroscopy is performed under local anaesthetic which is suitable for diagnostic arthroscopy but is more difficult for surgery. We use a continuous infusion of 3 litre bags of saline, a video screen and sterile camera. Using the technique of triangulation we view with a scope on one side and operate on the other side. The technique of direct arthroscopy is not frequently employed. The scope is inserted laterally and the operating instrument on the medial side. The surgery is then performed by reference to the video screen. What things can be seen through the scope? Folds of synovium or 'plica' are present in about 20% of the normal population and can give rise to symptoms. As a cause of pain they are probably over-diagnosed. Fraying of the meniscus may also be clinically insignificant. The lateral side is the best example of how good arthroscopy is at seeing around the back of a joint. A large lateral arthrotomy would not allow visualisation of the back of the joint. The patella is a difficult problem. Chondromalacia patellae should be diagnosed only after arthroscopy because it is only when there is macroscopic change in the patella that you can make the diagnosis. Anterior knee pain is common and is not synonymous with chondromalacia patellae. Other problems which may be seen apart from meniscal and cruciate tears are loose bodies, especially on the lateral side and popliteus tendonitis. When there is a tear of a large discoid meniscus an open menisectomy is justifiable because it is not easy to remove the whole tear through the arthroscope.

Of the knee joint ligament injuries, the most common is the medial ligament sprain. Usually it is superficial and recovers. Injuries of the deep part of the medial ligament create greater problems.

The famous O'Donoghue's triad with tears of medial ligament, medial meniscus and anterior cruciate ligament may arise. This is common in American footballers, a game which is designed to tear the knee and keep orthopaedic surgeons in business!

Most medial ligament injuries do recover without surgery, but the knee is not a simple hinged joint. The rotational element results in sportsmen who can run in a straight line but if they 'side-step' their knees may give out.

Blood in the joint indicates the severity of the injury. It is simple to ask the player: did the knee swell straight away or did it swell that night? If it swelled immediately then there has been a bleed. If it swells overnight it usually represents a synovial effusion. Up to 85% of haemarthroses in the knee are due to anterior-cruciate ligament tears. Other causes of bleeding include a peripheral tear of cartilage or an intra-articular fracture. The appearance of fat globules in the syringe indicates fracture. Aspiration of blood is a crucial aspect of management. The risks of infection have been exaggerated and we do it regularly, in casualty and in the clinics.

Anterior cruciate surgery is controversial. There are over 350 operations for reconstructing this ligament. There are the autologous grafts, using the patient's own tissue to reconstruct the ligament. A problem is that the tear is usually in mid substance and direct repair is like trying to sew two ends of a shaving brush.

There are extra-articular types of reconstruction, for example the transfer described by Slocome, where the insertion of the sartorius, gracilis and semi-tendinosus are utilised. These are flexors of the knee and this procedure attempts to tighten up the medial side of the knee and turn them into medial rotators.

The other extra-articular operation on the outside of the knee described by MacIntosh attempts to tighten the lateral side by taking a strip of fascia lata, re-routing it under the lateral ligament, and tying it back on itself. Good results are achieved with these operations but they tend to loosen in time, as do all procedures for anterior cruciate reconstruction. The Jones transfer takes a portion of patella tendon, leaving the tibial attachment, although that can be removed with a bone block and re-routed through. The problem with the femoral attachment in this procedure is the placement of the anterior cruciate ligament. Most orthopaedic surgeons now fix the femoral attachments with an 'over-the-top' procedure. However, rehabilitation is protracted. If the fixation fails on the femoral side, it can be difficult to salvage. David Jenkins in Cardiff contributed to the development of surgery with carbon fibre. This material acts as a scaffold for collagen formation. Experiments on sheep Achilles tendon with carbon fibre revealed collagen formation 6 months later.

Unfortunately carbon fibre can provoke intense synovitis in the joint. It is still used but is covered by the patient's own tissue (fascia lata) or as a composite ligament with a polyester covering.

The value of hamstring exercises in the management of anterior cruciate tears has been underestimated.

Discussion

BURRY: When I first started seeing sports players, surgery of the knee was haphazard with the surgeon triumphantly holding up a cartilage. By the time he got it out and discovered it was intact he was having to run his thumb-nail around to make a tear in the middle. There is no doubt that menisci were removed in error. Now we have a rational basis for surgery and there has been dramatic improvement in this aspect of medical care.

GIBSON: Would you agree that making a precise diagnosis on a clinical basis is extraordinarily difficult and if so, what are your criteria for arthroscopy?

WILLIAMS: Good question. Even though I did say history and examination is important it can be very difficult to make a diagnosis.

My criteria for arthroscopy include the classical injury in rugby football, where they have a twisting injury, they feel something goes on in their knee. We do not get that history in the UK as they do in the States. In the States, they say 'something popped in my knee'—so you know that is an anterior cruciate, but I don't get that history over in the UK, but they feel something has gone wrong in the knee—they have an effusion, overnight usually, and most injuries are to the medial meniscus although the lateral does certainly occur. You know there's always this conflict between medial ligament injuries and medial meniscal injuries, explained by the anatomy really, but a ligament injury is really posterior. Most medial meniscal injuries—even if it's a posterior horn, are often tender anteriorally, I find. I think the whole thing really depends on arthroscopy. Unfortunately there are waiting lists but luckily I do not have much of one because I am an enthusiast!

WALKDEN: Do you still do examination under anaesthesia before you put the scope in?

WILLIAMS: Yes, definitely—particularly for the anterior cruciate. As for the bucket-handle tear, 99% of locked knees straighten under anaesthetic. When you arthroscope you see the bucket-handle still in the intercondular notch but the locking is not mechanical.

HUGO: I wanted to ask—did I hear correctly?—that you've got a posterior cruciate that's torn, with a posterior displacement and you opted for no surgery? As a South African I wonder how much better you may have played in 1974 without the tear.

WILLIAMS: Well, I can tell you the scenario about my knee. I have problems with my knee and I think that probably my patellar osteoarthritis is due to instability of my knee. Now, here comes the argument—do you prophylactically replace someone's ligament? I don't regret my decision at all, and I would do the same again. My problems may have been a result of not having an operation but I did not want to have huge surgery.

BURRY: John, we are actually talking aloof to the fact that people begin to neglect their hamstring as being the stabilizers of the torn anterior cruciate. There are some papers which suggest that conservative management by remedial exercise in a rehabilitative phase has a result not too inferior to surgery.

WILLIAMS: Absolutely. I always send my patients for intensive physiotherapy. If that does not do it then we discuss the pros and cons of surgery. But that is the important thing—you have got to have a motivated person. The best result I have ever had was a Welsh international hooker who played in the Welsh Cup Final 9 months after anterior cruciate surgery. But, again he is not a three-quarter. A three-quarter needs the speed more than a front-row forward. So, you know the most important thing is to discuss the pros and cons, and are they going to work on the rehabilitation? I agree with you—we've got two ex-Welsh internationals who have incredible clinical instability, their knees wobble forward, as does mine, but functionally they are fine. As with the ankle, re-education of proprioceptors is important.

BURRY: A case in point was a gentleman who played quite well for New Zealand for a number of years and I remember having to examine him when he came with the All-Blacks 1971 tour, after he sprained his ankle. I went to examine his foot and it virtually came away in my hand. I put it back on again hurriedly! The knee was not too hot either it just wobbled about and yet functionally he was 'A1'. I said to him: 'how long have your foot and ankle been like this?' He said: 'Oh years, it doesn't worry me too much'.

DAVIES: In partially torn anterior cruciate ligaments, how do you manage those? Do they exist?

WILLIAMS: The answer is yes, they do exist, because they are separate bundles, actually. Most of them do well conservatively. It is usually a total tear of the ligament which sometimes needs surgery.

O'BRIEN: Can I just add that muscle strengthening prior to surgery is also very important—it will really speed up the rehabilitation of the patients, especially if you start it at least 2 weeks prior to the surgery of a fit athlete.

WILLIAMS: That is another good reason—I send them all for the treatment before—there are some which I think are going to come to surgery. It is important to build the muscles up before surgery.

ENGLISH QUESTIONER: Just an interesting story about a local chap I saw—a rugby player just recently—who happened to ask me in passing why his left knee was feeling a bit loose. So I had a look at him and at first sight it looked like he had a positive anterior drawer sign. Of course I looked from the side before pulling the tibia forward and it was quite obvious he had a sort of marked depression of the tibia, already being in a backward position. I asked him whether he had any history of injury at all—he had no prior trauma, no effusions, nothing whatsoever, but he quite clearly had a totally absent posterior cruciate ligament. Have you ever come across that?

WILLIAMS: Certainly, it's fairly well documented that you may have congenital absence of the cruciate ligament. Usually it is bilateral and that is why it is important to examine the normal joint as well.

11: Rehabilitation of the Injured Player: an Overview

H.C.BURRY

THE GAME in which we are involved is a game which confines 30 large muddy players to a prescribed space and due to the nature of the contest of pursuing a piece of soggy pigskin around a wet paddock, we end up, inevitably with injuries.

We cannot distinguish acute medical care from rehabilitation which must start on the first day. For example, a player may present with a large haemarthrosis a week after injury and with wasting of the quadriceps. Extra medical care and attention is then required, merely because of neglect. Rehabilitation should start on day 1.

Another example might be the back of the thigh where a large dent represents a mass of scar tissue adherent to surrounding tissues. On running, another tear occurs and the player is told to rest until pain-free. This is a neglected soft tissue injury and the sort of consequence that rehabilitation attempts to avoid.

Evaluation is the key to rehabilitation and involves more than just a diagnosis. One has to look at the functional loss and what that means to the person. Sensory loss is uncommon in rugby injuries, but the possibility of perceptual and cognitive functional loss, as in head injuries together with the psychological effects of injury are more common. We have to try and put ourselves in the position of the injured player and try to see what it looks like from his or her perspective.

Rehabilitation: an Overview

One of the problems of medicine is the model of injury; disease or ageing produces pathology, pain and dysfunction. Treatment equals cure except that there is the odd recalcitrant who fails. When pain and dysfunction develop there is concomitant anxiety. The anxiety will lead to tension and the tension itself will cause pain and dysfunction. A vicious circle can easily develop whereby the unwary physician or surgeon will give more and more treatments under the misconception that the original pathology still exists. The original precipitating pathology may have disappeared and the effects of anxiety taken over. More referrals, investigations and surgery will have a disastrous effect.

Once a diagnosis is established, a plan needs to be devised, like any other business venture. Rather than merely saying: 'I'll treat you with physiotherapy and hopefully you'll be alright', you have to say that this man has function loss and what is a realistic goal? Can he be ready in 1 week, or 1 month? Is it appropriate to have him running by the end of the first week, running with the team within 2 weeks, and back in competition in 4? One needs to identify a realistic goal and work out the strategies required to reach that goal.

One needs to restore strength, stamina, function and suppleness to joints. A man experiencing back pain may be immensely strong and yet be unable to do sit-up exercises because in all his training he had neglected the fact that there are two aspects to the control of the spine; the paraspinal muscles that people always identify with the back, and the often forgotten abdominal muscles. An appropriate programme in his instance would be to restore abdominal muscle strength and function, and ensure balance between agonists and antagonists.

To obtain suppleness as well as stamina and strength, players may benefit from attending ballet school. The psychology of the patient is important. There is a group who have a fear of not being able to cope, who tell the doctor not to hesitate to tell them they are out for the season. One needs to understand and help to confront the challenge that is before them. If they turn their back on it they may never forgive themselves. At the other extreme, one may be confronted by a player who has had multiple injuries yet is determined to carry on. One such person was a 35-year-old rugby hooker. His neck was a shambles and he had osteoarthritic knees, and one shoulder had huge osteophytes. I said rather doubtfully, not knowing how to approach the subject: 'Have you ever thought of retiring?' His body system was past rehabilitation, and resurrection was his only hope!

There are three Cs in rehabilitation; communication, between various parties; co-ordination of programmes; and co-operation. It is important to identify the patient's advocate who will ensure it all happens. In some circumstances that person could be the coach who can become a key person in rehabilitation by supervising the exercise programme, ensuring a gradual return to full function, and making sure an accurate assessment is done by appropriately skilled staff before competition is resumed.

12: Application of Isokinetic Studies to Sporting Injuries

MOIRA O'BRIEN

ISOKINETIC machines represent a new era in the assessment and rehabilitation of injuries. They can assess different muscle actions [1]. Isometric action occurs when tension is produced, but there is no change in length; this causes the least stress on the muscle. Concentric action is when the muscle shortens as it produces tension, and eccentric action occurs when it lengthens [2]. The latter produces the greatest stress on the muscle, but is the most powerful action of the muscle. From the rehabilitation point of view, this is vital because as isometric contraction produces the least tension, it should be used first in any rehabilitation programme.

Isokinetic machines provide an accommodating resistance at a dynamic present speed, so that there is maximum resistance at each point within the range of motion, unlike isotonic exercise, where the amount of weight used may be limited by the weakest point in the range of motion [3]. Isokinetic machines keep the speed constant, but the resistance varies and matches the force applied to the lever. The speed, amount of force and the range of motion can be predetermined in many isokinetic machines on the market. Some of the machines can only test or rehabilitate in the concentric mode, while others can also test in the eccentric phase, which is the most useful for diagnostic and research protocols [4,5].

Isokinetic machines test muscle groups acting on a joint, not individual muscles. Some of the computerised equipment can test in the isometric and isotonic, as well as the isokinetic mode. These are more expensive, but more suitable for research and diagnosis [2].

The unit of measurement is newton-meters. Power is measured in newton-meters and the torque, or moment, is a measure of the effectiveness of the force, in producing rotation around an axis. It is important to know the axis of the joint and the torque that is required. An important aspect of setting up these machines is to realise that they require knowledge of the joints and muscles involved and that calibration takes time; it takes a minimum of 30 minutes for the machine to warm up and then the patient has to be correctly positioned; the test itself takes relatively little time.

Most joints in the body are polycentric and the machine axis has to be aligned with the optimum part of the joint being tested. The position of the patient is also important, so that in testing the knee joint, one needs to know which plane is required [5]. One can examine it in two positions, sitting or prone [6]. In the sitting position one can only test from 0 to 90° of flexion. A wider range requires the patient to be prone. This is important when testing for patellofemoral pain, because pain may not occur in the sitting position, but may only occur at 130° of flexion [7].

When testing muscles acting on a joint, you must stabilise the proximal joint [8]. Standardisation is a problem, as the centre of rotation of most joints are not fixed, they vary with the different positions of the joint. To standardise testing, you must use the same agreed axis each time. Some people use the joint line, others the fibular head for testing the knee. The true axis is the femoral epicondyle.

One must also correct for gravity and this is done automatically in some machines. One cannot compare one limb of a very light-weight person with that of a heavy person. Note must be made of whether patients wear shoes. The age, sex, weight and the level of physical activity must be recorded, whether before or after injury, and whether in the early or late part of the season.

It is important to have a definite protocol to warm up the muscles before testing, because the patient's muscles must be warmed beforehand. The patient must be told what is going to happen, and there should be a practice run at the speeds that will be involved. It is essential to prevent hyperextension of a joint, particularly if you have to recalibrate.

A medical history is valuable because if one tests the upper limbs in the isometric mode, there is a much greater increase in blood pressure.

For diagnostic purposes at least two speeds should be used, 30° and 120° per second; a third speed of 180° per second may be used for athletes. Each speed should be tested concentrically and eccentrically. The shape of the curve should be observed. The hamstrings and quadriceps have totally different curves [9]. The former should have a smooth curve, increasing from 0 to 90°. The eccentric curve is higher than the concentric. Not only is it important to look at the shape of the curve but also the newton-meters produced, because a decrease occurs in anterior cruciate tears and other ligament injuries [10].

At slow speeds, the concentric action of the hamstrings is 60% of the concentric action of the quadriceps. As the speed increases this ratio diminishes. In everyday life, the eccentric action of the hamstrings often counteracts the concentric action of the quadriceps, e.g. at the end of the swing phase of walking, the concentric action of the quadriceps is opposed by the eccentric action of the hamstrings, and these should be nearly equal. So it is the ratio of the eccentric hamstrings that should be compared with the concentric quadriceps. The eccentric phase is the most useful from the diagnostic point of view.

When testing the knee, the maximum load on the patella occurs at an angle of 45°. At slower speeds, loading lasts for a longer period of time, which may cause pain. The higher the load the greater the pain.

The torque curve for the quadriceps should be a smooth curve which increases from 0 to 90°. In patients with knee pain, a break phenomenon may be observed. It only occurs in the eccentric phase of the quadriceps and is more marked at slow speeds. It is closely related to pain. The break usually occurs at an angle of 45°, a drop of 5 newton-meters is a break [6]. It is postulated that maximal loading causes a neural reflex inhibiting quadriceps contraction, and it takes 10° to recover, then the curve starts to take off again. If a patient with knee pain, who has no patella pain or a break in the slow, eccentric, quadriceps graph in the sitting position, he may develop pain and the break phenomenon at an angle of 130° when testing in the prone position.

The power or endurance of a muscle group may be tested by doing repetitive movements. One can actually see at which range of movement the patient has the greatest power, or which is the weakest. From this information, one can estimate whether it is the concentric or eccentric phase which requires the greater rehabilitation.

To rehabilitate, one must improve the concentric force of the quads and maintain the antagonistic, eccentric, strength of the hamstrings. One side can be compared with the other and different joints can be evaluated, and it can also be used in training. Reliability, repeatability and safety measures are essential [11].

The oblique portion of the abdominal muscles play an important role in supporting the lumbar spine; it is not possible to assess them in most isokinetic machines. When one buys a machine it is important to know its capabilities and whether it will be used in diagnosis or rehabilitation or both.

Discussion

BATH DOCTOR: Am I right in thinking that concentric–eccentric ratio requirements may be different in the different sports, such as rugby?

O'BRIEN: The concentric–eccentric ratio of the different muscle groups varies, depending on the sport and the type of work that is done. During the phases of the gait cycle, the relationship between the hamstrings and the quadriceps changes. At the end of the swing phase the quadriceps is contracting concentrically, while the hamstrings action is eccentric to prevent excessive extension of the knee. At other times both are acting together concentrically.

GIBSON: Is this machine being evaluated in a controlled way therapeutically?

O'BRIEN: I can give you references. We only use it for diagnosis, but in America, Australia and Israel it is used in rehabilitation. Brian Edwards of Perth, Western Australia, has a spinal injuries rehabilitation programme for low back pain. He is working on a group of people who have been out of work for at least 6 months. They are using the KinCom as part of a comprehensive programme with very good results. Using the KinCom you can demonstrate at which range of movement the muscles are weakest, and one can improve on this. Previously only manual testing was available for assessment.

BURRY: But I must say that I am not totally persuaded. We have got the equipment and we have got research workers using it at the moment and reviewing the literature. Really it is still, I do not think, totally persuasive. I think a lot more work needs to be done for validation, which is really why we have got to see whether there is anything in it.

In Australia it costs about 80 000 dollars for the basic equipment, which is a lot of money to spend unless you know for sure that it is going to be valuable and therapeutic. Certainly I have no doubt that it has psychotherapeutic value. People can get a print-out of what they have achieved and how much power has been generated, and so on. I think from a research point of view as you correctly say, to be able to get a print-out of power through a whole range of movements may isolate a weakness at one end or the other of the scale.

GILFEATHER: Moira, could you please go over again the importance you attach to the development of abdominal muscles in people with back problems?

O'BRIEN: Yes, one of the most important factors in back problems is that a lot of these people have very poor abdominal muscles. One of the most important adverse factors in people with low back pain is that they very often have very poor abdominal muscles, and a large number are doing the wrong type of exercises. They are doing fast sit-ups, often with their feet held. They have very strong psoas muscles, but poor abdominals. Exercises to improve the abdominals must include the upper, lower and the obliques. The role of the abdominals in most sports is to contract isometrically to maintain intra-abdominal pressure and so help to splint the spine, in some sports they act eccentrically and this may occasionally occur in rugby.

To improve the upper abdominal muscles, the subject lies on his back with bent knees, feet on the ground *not held*. Hands on chest, the subject comes up slowly, to approximately 45°, holds this position for 10, then goes back slowly. For the lower abdominals, if they are very weak, the person lies on the back, both knees bent, brings the two knees onto the anterior abdominal wall slowly, and then lets them down slowly, gradually increasing the number of repetitions until they can do 25 easily. Then lying on their back, with one knee bent, the other leg straight, lift the straight leg vertically upwards by contracting the lower abdominals, so that the buttock is raised from the floor. Again, gradually increase the number of times, till it can be repeated 25 times on both sides, then progress to lifting both bent knees vertically upwards 2 or 3 inches.

To improve the obliques, in the same position as for the upper abdominals, both arms out straight, bring the right arm to the outer part of the left knee, and hold for 10. Then go back slowly. When this can be done 25 times, place the heel of the right foot on the left knee, with the hands around the lower part of the neck and the elbows together, so that the neck cannot be pulled forwards. Bring the left elbow to the right knee, hold for 10, then go back slowly; gradually increase till this can be done 25 times. Throwing and catching a medicine ball is also a good exercise.

References

1 Farrell M, Richards JG. Analysis of the reliability and validity of the kinetic communicator device. *Med Sci Sport Exer* 1986; **18**: 44–9.
2 Hakkinen K, Komi PV, Tesch P. Effect of combined concentric and eccentric strength training and detraining on force–time muscle fibre, and metabolic characteristics of leg extensor muscles. *Scand J Sports Sci* 1981; **3**: 50–8.
3 Stauber WT. Measurement of muscle function in man. In: Grisogono V, ed. *Sports Injuries*. New York: Churchill Livingstone, 187–212.
4 Rothstein JM. Measurement and clinical practice. Theory and applications. In: Rothstein JM, ed. *Measurement in Physical Therapy: Clinics in Physical Therapy*. New York: Churchill Livingstone, 1985: 10.
5 Marshall RN, Taylor AS. The skeletal muscle force–velocity relationships. 1. Its significance and its measurement. *NZ J Sports Med* 1990; Autumn: 8–10.

6 Worrel TW, Denegar CR, Armstrong SL. Effect of body position on hamstring muscle group average torque. *J Orth Sports Phys Ther* 1990; **11**: 449–52.
7 Dvir Z, Shklar A, Halperin N *et al*. Concentric and eccentric torque variations of the quadriceps femoris in patellofemoral pain syndrome. *Clin Biomech* 1990; **5**.
8 Hart DL, Stobbe TJ, Till CW. Effect of trunk stabilization on quadriceps femoris muscle torque. *Phys Ther* 1984; **64**: 1375–80.
9 Wyatt MP, Edwards AM. Comparison of quadriceps and hamstring torque values during isokinetic exercise. *J Orth Sports Phys Ther* 1980; **60**: 412–19.
10 Kannus P. Ratio of hamstring to quadriceps muscles, strength in the anterior cruciate ligament: relationship to long term recovery. *Phys Ther* 1988; **68**: 961–5.
11 Taylor NAS, McNair PJ, Stanley SN *et al*. The skeletal muscle force–velocity relationship. 2. Its application in functional assessment for training and rehabilitation. *NZ J Sports Med* 1990; Winter: 28–33.

13: The Management of Soft Tissue Injuries

C.HAMMOND

THE FIRST thing to consider is the aetiology of soft tissue injury [1–4]; is it acute or chronic? The chronic injury usually occurs in endurance athletes, the acute injury in explosive athletes, direct and indirect. In rugby the whole gamut occurs because it is a game that is partly endurance, partly explosive and injury can arise directly or indirectly because it is a body contact sport.

Knowing how an injury has arisen may help to prevent it in the future. If a player arrives late and in the first quarter of the game pulls a hamstring, it is clear that he has gone cold onto the field. If a forward has a hamstring tear in the last quarter of the game, the chances are that he is not fit enough.

The first aim of rehabilitation is an accurate diagnosis. One then has to provide the most favourable conditions for healing, following which strengthening the tissue to its maximum strength receives priority. In chronic injuries this should be emphasised because the tissue has broken down through weakness.

Injury severity can be classified as grades 1, 2 and 3 [1–4]. Grade 1 is less than 5% of the tissues involved; such players hardly ever stop during the game and feel pain only after leaving the field. These may miss one game and receive minor physiotherapy. In grade 2 there is 5–50% fibre tear. Players invariably leave the field with pain: there is local tenderness and on stress have moderate to severe pain. Grade 3 implies 50–100% fibre tear, symptoms are similar to grade 2 but more exaggerated. The major difference is loss of function but paradoxically players do not complain of pain on stressing the lesion due to loss of continuity of tissue. It is vital to distinguish grades 2 and 3 because grade 3 almost always requires surgery. A ruptured Achilles tendon which is missed for 1 week is difficult to repair. Equally, a complete rupture of a medial knee ligament may be complicated by granulation tissue if repair is delayed.

In acute soft tissue trauma there are three distinct pathological phases [1,5]. Phase 1 which lasts up to 72 hours is a simple, non-specific inflammatory condition. There is a humoral and cellular element involving prostaglandins (PG), E1 and E2, and granulocytes. The release of PG increases permeability of capillary membranes which causes the swelling and produces pain. Anti-inflammatory drugs exert an effect at this phase [1,3]. These may be taken orally although topical non-steroidal anti-inflammatory agents such as felbinac (Traxam) have an undoubted role.

Phase 2 is the repair phase which is when collagen is produced. Production of collagen starts 48–72 hours after the acute inflammatory stage and in the initial repair phase, quantity exceeds quality. Phase 3 is the remodelling phase which is a continuation and blends into repair phase and continues for up to 6 months. Understanding this phase is the crux of rehabilitation. It is at this point that the tensile strength of the collagen is increased to match the direction and degree of stress to which it is subjected. Thus, early mobility and stress on reparative collagen is essential and should start from 48–72 hours after the injury and continue progressively until full strength is attained.

There is no place for the injection of steroids in acute injury: it inhibits the early stages of collagen formation and reduces its subsequent tensile strength [1,2,6].

Practical management

Early treatment (48–72 hours) of the acute phase follows the acronym of 'RICE'—rest, ice [7–10], compression, elevation. Ice chips are preferred to any other coolant [11]. Studies show varying temperature drop in the tissues relative to time applied but in that vasoconstriction occurs up to 25°C and cold vasodilatation below 25°C [12], it is counterproductive to apply ice for too long—10–30 minutes, three or four times a day is sufficient.

In the pathological repair phase—from 48–72 hours onwards—stress must be applied to realign the newly formed collagen and maximise the tensile strength [1]. Early mobility is therefore essential and the amount carefully monitored—rehabilitating is an art and not a science and a good physiotherapist is invaluable. Too cautious an approach can leave the patient still disabled at 6 weeks, too aggressive an approach may produce further damage. Limits of pain are the guidelines but because they are subjective, the severity of pain as perceived by the patient must be gauged against the nature of the injury. Non-weight bearing mobility exercises are used initially progressing through isometric to isotonic with progressive resistance to maximum strength. Full strength and mobility must be achieved before return to sport.

In addition to early mobility and controlled progressive strength programme there are three additional points of emphasis:

1 It is vital when rehabilitating damaged tissue that aerobic strength is maintained;

2 In the knee and ankle it is crucial for proprioception to be rehabilitated as well as strength; and

3 There is one exception to the aggressive approach—a large quadriceps haematoma should be treated with rest far beyond what is recommended for other lesions to avoid myositis ossificans.

Discussion

DAVIES: How do you help your athletes to define pain? You say exercise within the limits of pain.

HAMMOND: Yes I do. What I usually say is: 'I want you to tell me when there is discomfort'. So we try to stretch them to the point of discomfort but not pain. For the collagen to be remodelled correctly it has to be done. The main problem is what the patient thinks is discomfort and what I think is discomfort—knowing your patient is a great help!

References

1 Oakes BW. Acute soft tissue injuries: nature and management. *Aust Fam Physician* 1981; **10**(suppl): 3–16.

2 Zarens B. Soft tissue injury and repair—biomechanical aspects. *Int J Sports Med* 1982; **3**(suppl): 9–11.

3 Muckle DS. Injuries in sport. *Roy Soc Health J* 1982; **102**: 93–4.

4 Garrick JG. The sports medicine patient. *Nursing Clin N Am* 1981; **16**: 759–66.

5 Van der Meulin JHC. Present state of knowledge on processes of healing in collagen structures. *Int J Sports Med* 1982; **3**: 4–8.

6 Bentley S. The treatment of sports injuries by local injections. *Br J Sports Med* 1981; **15**: 71–4.

7 Basur RL, Shepherd E, Mouzas GL. A cooling method in the treatment of ankle strain. *Practitioner* 1976; 708.

8 Hocutt JE, Jaffe R, Rylander CR, Beebe JK. Cryotherapy in ankle sprains. *Am J Sports Med* 1982; **10**: 316–19.

9 Kalenak A, Medlar CE, Fleagle SB, Hochberg WJ. Athletic injuries: heat versus cold. *Am Fam Physician* 1975; **12**: 131–4.

10 Starkey JA. The treatment of ankle sprains by simultaneous use of intermittent compression and ice packs. *Am J Sports Med* 1976; **4**: 142–4.

11 McMasters WC, Liddle S, Waugh TR. Laboratory evaluation of various cold therapy methods. *Med Sci Sports* 1976; **8**: 39–42.

12 Pappenheimer SL, Eversole SL, Sotorivera A. Vascular responses to temperature changes in isolated perfused hindlimbs of the cat. *Am J Physiol* 1948; **155**: 458.

14: Podiatry in Rehabilitation and Acute Rehabilitation Management

J.E.DAVIES

THE PODIATRIST is an important member of the rehabilitation team. In the USA, podiatry has been a recognised skill for a long time and podiatrists tend to divide into two groups: (a) the surgical who operate on the fore- and mid-foot; and (b) the biomechanical. Many of the chronic over-use injuries affecting the lower limbs such as shin splints, the iliotibial tract syndrome and anterior knee pain, etc., are due to foot imbalances. From this point of view, the podiatrist is an integral part of sports injury management. In rugby, boot manufacture is a multi-million dollar industry. There is much work to be done in this particular area. The American grid iron football looked at the multi-cleated boot many years ago. In rugby, with playing surfaces improving, new stadia being built, it will be interesting to see what developments occur in relation to boot design.

Specific joint assessments may be made of the feet, for example the sub-talar joint in the neutral position. Of the total range of movement, two-thirds is inversion, as measured from the leg, and a third is eversion. Forefoot imbalances can be assessed with a forefoot measuring device. What the podiatrist can then do is introduce padding and strapping which is applied to simulate the effect of an orthotic. The patient's gait is then reassessed on a treadmill. After padding and strapping, given some time of trial, the foot is then casted using plaster of Paris from which any type of orthosis can be made to compensate for any intrinsic foot length or back imbalance previously assessed.

There are approximately 40 different types of insoles and orthoses available for a variety of sporting activities. Podiatrists will advise on the specific types of running or sporting shoe from the plethora of designs available. The correct selection of orthoses and shoes is very much an integral part of the correct mechanical and biomechanical management.

In Wales there is a rehabilitation centre with these modalities as well as isokinetics, a gait analysis unit and hydrotherapy. The Welsh Rugby Union has insured all the national squad players and they can utilise this private rehabilitation centre.

15: Is There a Risk of Developing Osteoarthritis Through Sport?

T.GIBSON

ALL ELDER statesmen in rugby should think about osteoarthritis (OA) from time to time. There is a consensus that regular sporting activity, with some exceptions, hardly ever leads to OA or precocious degeneration of joints. It is conceivable that this optimism is misplaced as is plain from a critical analysis of the studies quoted to sustain this view.

Common sense seems to tell us that specific joints exposed to frequent stress might well lead to premature degeneration. In certain occupations, areas of the spine or peripheral joints which are regularly exposed to vigorous use can be susceptible to OA, both radiological and symptomatic. We know that miners are more likely than the rest of the population to develop OA of the elbows and knees, and in the same way pneumatic drillers and dockers, OA of other sites [1,2]. It follows from that simple observation that sportsmen who regularly expose and stress particular joints may hypothetically develop OA.

There are many largely anecdotal series of specific patterns of OA associated with particular sports; cricketers who expose their fingers to regular trauma; wrestlers are prone to OA of the spine; boxers, especially those who sustain fractures near joints may develop OA at carpometacarpal sites. It has also been claimed that baseball pitchers may develop changes in the shoulder, an unusual joint for the development of OA.

Radiological changes do not necessarily imply symptoms or disability. There have been numbers of claims made, based entirely on X-ray appearance. Vincelette *et al.* [3] claimed that severe radiological OA occurred in North American football players, and the abnormality was seen in the ankles and the hindfoot. These X-ray changes were principally of sclerosis and what looked like large osteophytes. Klunder *et al.* [4] more recently described degenerative changes in the hips amounting to sclerosis and osteophytosis. There are two other studies, one as recently as 1989, where radiological changes have been given undue emphasis [5,6].

With the exception of Klunder *et al.* [4], none of the above authors mentioned symptoms or signs. We all accept that with increasing age, what are sometimes presumed to represent degenerative change may occur in the cervical spine. For example, over the age of 55, at least half of all people have narrowing of the disc spaces and osteophytes in the absence of symptoms [7]. Around the knee joint, it is common to see the development of osteophytes with ageing but in the absence of joint space narrowing. The unwary could easily attribute such changes to OA in the clinical sense. Although X-ray changes of degeneration may be unaccompanied by symptoms, the converse is also true. One may see symptoms which are in no way related to the radiological changes. For example, X-ray cystic changes in the talus were unrelated to a patient's ankle pain which was due to tenosynovitis (Fig. 15.1). Apart from the ankle and hindfoot in North American football already alluded to, there have been a number of other studies involving soccer and running (cross-country and long distance but not sprinting). In some of these it has been claimed that OA is an outcome and in others not at all [4,8–12]. These are often quoted in surveys of joint disease in athletes. Their deficiencies include the smallness of the numbers. The largest was a study of the hip involving 74 champion runners [12]. It is impossible to form firm conclusions on the basis of such sample sizes. Another problem is age. In the study by Vincelette *et al.* [3] the average age was 23. What is more, all participants were still playing American football. It is absurd to make the claim that OA of the ankle and hindfoot is a regular occurrence in players who have no symptoms, who are young and still playing. The crucial question is whether OA in sports people is advanced by a decade or so. One needs to look at people aged 60–80 years.

An obvious way of trying to examine this question is to see whether sports people are over-represented amongst those who are coming to surgery for joint replacement. There has been one study which has looked at the problem in this fashion. This was a relatively small survey of 100

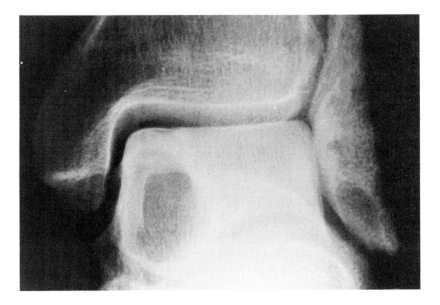

Fig. 15.1 Cyst in talus of a patient with tenosynovitis. The cyst did not cause the symptoms.

patients scheduled for total hip replacement [13]. The author claimed that sports people were not over-represented. The ex-sports people in the population were not examined in any other way and it is impossible to say whether they were younger, or whether any particular sport predominated. There is scope for more work to be conducted along these lines.

In body contact sports, and indeed in some other athletic pursuits, it is the knee which is particularly vulnerable to injury. It is in the population with a history of knee injury that one might find precocious OA. One of the best studies of knee ligament injuries was written by Balfors [14]. He noted that of the whole series, 10% were incapacitated, in the sense that in due course they had to change or modify work or had to give up their sport. In this study population, clinical and radiological OA was apparent in 7%. It is interesting that he distinguished the mere development of osteophytosis, which appeared in about a third. The striking observation and one which has become universally accepted is that OA was confined to those patients who had undergone meniscectomy. It is almost exclusively in this group of patients that OA is regularly seen. The other worthwhile observation of this study was that posterior, anterior and collateral ligamentous injuries were included and some were treated conservatively. In no instance was OA an outcome except when associated with removal of the cartilage.

Are there any other factors associated with a cartilage tear which are important and which may influence or contribute to the development of OA? In a study by Muckle [15] it was claimed that in those patients who had a clear history of locking, who had associated ligamentous injury, involvement of the lateral meniscus, a peripheral tear, delayed surgery or if there were a chronic post-operative effusion the circumstances militated against a successful outcome in the long term. Some of these points have been confirmed by other observers more recently. It certainly seems likely that damage and removal of the lateral meniscus is much more injurious than medial meniscal tears. If it is true that some of these factors are operative, it raises a question about the refinements which have been introduced by orthopaedic surgeons in the management of meniscal tears.

The prevalent view is that by a piecemeal approach and operation through the arthroscope, the development of OA is something that we are going to see much less of. I am not familiar with any study which has actually demonstrated beyond doubt that the outcome of OA is less prevalent using modern surgical techniques. It is hopeful, and there are sound hypothetical reasons for believing that is likely, but the wholesale use of such procedures has not been performed for long enough for sound judgement. If it is true that numbers of other factors, like the site of the lesion and the period before surgical intervention, are important in the subsequent development of OA then it may well be that we shall continue to see, perhaps on a smaller scale, late development of OA in people treated by modern techniques.

The diagnosis of knee pain is extraordinarily difficult. In a study of 129 chronic knee pain patients (knee pain of more than 8 weeks duration) we found that it was difficult to make a clinical diagnosis of a torn meniscus, or indeed of any other particular pathology [16]. For example, in our population of patients who were subsequently shown to have meniscal tears on arthroscopy, only 59% had an obviously acute injury. Patients who had characteristic histories and typical findings, not infrequently had normal arthroscopy. Patients who had pain of insidious onset and atypical findings not infrequently were found to have meniscal tears.

Amongst the conclusions that we drew from this study was that arthroscopy should be much more readily available in the UK. It is a resource which is not always accessible and treating athletes with knee pain who do not have an obvious acute injury or a persistent effusion, can be inappropriately protracted. Other means of investigation, such as magnetic resonance imaging (MRI) and arthrography are not as sensitive at establishing the cause. If it is true that the longer the delay between operative intervention and injury the more likely the development of OA,

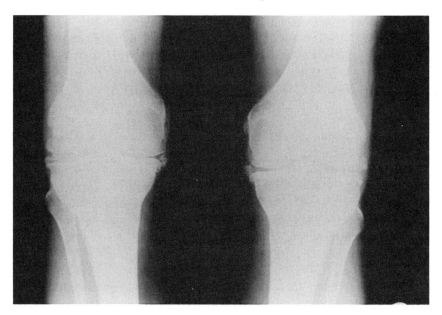

Fig. 15.2 Knee X-ray of a patient who has had meniscectomy of both knees and subsequently developed osteoarthritis and chondrocalcinosis (calcification of cartilage).

delayed access to arthroscopy becomes an important ethical or even political issue.

The cause of the OA that follows meniscectomy is uncertain. It is presumed that damage is done to the hyaline cartilage in the removal of the meniscus, or perhaps in the period prior to that and that some incongruity or pitting of the cartilage surface takes place. Another phenomenon in meniscectomy patients followed up for a sufficient time is chondrocalcinosis (Fig. 15.2). In one series it occurred in 20% overall; in 6% of those aged less than 50 and in almost a third of those aged more than 65 [17]. These patients were much more likely to be symptomatic in terms of stiffness, effusion and recurrent acute arthritis. They also had more severe OA.

The presumption is, although it is difficult to know which is 'chicken' and which is 'egg', that calcium pyrophosphate crystals accumulate in the cartilage, and which may be liberated from time to time, may be causing recurrent injury through the release of lysosomes and other proteolytic enzymes liberated during inflammation. It would be interesting to see whether this phenomena is also apparent in patients who are treated by modern surgical techniques.

[85]

Attempts by orthopaedic surgeons to preserve as much cartilage as possible at meniscectomy are based on sound hypothetical reasons. A study published in 1981 looked at 115 cadavers and it was noted that more than half, many of whom had succumbed to trauma but a majority of whom had simply died of natural causes had some sort of meniscal problem [18]. This was manifest as fragmentation or small tears and in such people there seemed to be no relationship at all to OA. These authors concluded that the retention of small areas of meniscus could have a protective effect on cartilage.

The literature contains additional hypotheses and associations about OA and sport. The work by Murray and Duncan [19] defined a problem which they termed 'epiphysiolysis'. Abnormal angulation of the femoral head was followed by precocious OA in people who in adolescence or childhood had been enthusiastically athletic. This was a series of elegant studies which have never been refuted.

The question of anterior knee pain is so often the bane of athletic injury clinics. The expression incorporates the pathological change of chondromalacia patellae. It is accepted that anterior knee pain is not the prelude to OA, although there are still orthopaedic surgeons who take a different view. In an athletic injury clinic, rugby players may account for about 50% of such patients [20]. However, it is runners who are especially susceptible. The age distribution of such patients makes it clear that it is a problem which evolves and resolves in the course of time in the vast majority. It is worth commenting that despite at least one optimistic editorial in the *British Medical Journal* [21] it is not a condition that resolves in a year or two and it may become a chronic problem [22]. It has been argued that in that small number who have indefinite retropatellar discomfort which began in mid-life, one is dealing with a pathology that leads to OA of the patellofemoral joint.

Osteochondritis dissecans of the knee or ankle is a condition that may lead to OA (Fig. 15.3). If there is subsequent incongruity of the cartilage there is filling in and healing. What advice do we give to young people who are keen on sports, who have osteochrondritis dissecans? There are no clear guide-lines because such people are soon asymptomatic. Should one advise such people never to play sport? The probability is that they are vulnerable to OA. Do we know whether playing sport increases the risk or is it something that exists irrespective of how they conduct their lives?

Chronic effusions and haemarthroses may also predispose to OA. There are theoretical reasons why persistent effusions will do so by virtue of ligamentous stretching, laxity and an element of subsequent joint instability. Recurrent or persistent haemarthrosis may be injurious to cartilage by

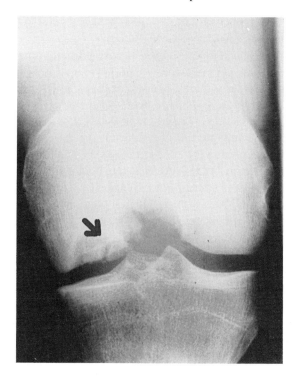

Fig. 15.3 X-ray of knee showing severe osteochondritis dissecans.

evoking a local inflammatory response. An extreme example is haemophilia, where recurrent bleeds into a joint may cause devastating change. A major problem of haemophiliac patients by virtue of their relative longevity, is joint damage of the ankles and knees. These are often joints which have not been exposed to any particular trauma but which have been the site of recurrent bleeds. There is good reason for aspirating haemarthroses whenever we see them.

Those who take regular exercise are less susceptible to osteoporosis and bone mass measurements show that the density of not only the spine but also the peripheral skeleton may be increased. Another hypothetical point is that increased bone density, hardening of bone, especially near a joint may increase susceptibility to OA [10].

There are those who seriously believe that people with hyper-mobile joints are not only prone to injury but also to OA in later life. It is not an argument that has been pursued vigorously, nor one which is held with total conviction, but there are theoretical reasons for suspecting that such an association might exist. From the practical standpoint, what should one do about people who want to play body contact sports and who have marked hyper-mobility?

OA in sports people is a topic which has lain dormant for some time but has been revived by the availability of markers for joint damage. Keratan sulphate may be measured in the serum or urine. In OA and rheumatoid disease it is thought that it may be indicative of active joint damage and it is an obvious parameter to measure in athletes. It is difficult to be sure whether markers really do reflect significant damage but some relevant observations have been made. Measurements in a marathon runner who ran three marathons in 3 days revealed elevation of keratan sulphate over the following days [23]. This is prima-facie evidence of damaged cartilage. Keratan sulphate is released into the circulation at the time of cartilage repair. Pyridinoline is a different marker which is enjoying popularity in the investigation of rheumatic diseases. It is a protein which cross-links collagen in the cartilage and is measurable in the urine. It may indicate joint damage. In a study that was performed in people who were participating in a run and walk of 33 miles in the Pennines, more runners had positive results, indicating some sort of metabolic change to their cartilage [24]. One runner had an exceptionally high level. These observations have again prompted the discussion of whether vigorous athletic endeavour may induce changes in joint cartilage which may, in turn, at some time lead to OA.

The consensus is that for those who pretend to enjoy running before breakfast, the likelihood of developing OA is remote. It is important to realise that one cannot extrapolate from one sport to another. One must not be lulled into a false sense of security because there have been eight studies of people who run, the majority of which have seemed to show that there is no risk at all of developing OA. Rugby is conspicuous amongst sports in not having been the subject of such study. Before one can be entirely optimistic about the impact of this activity on the joints there is a need to do the right sort of studies.

References

1 Kellgren J, Lawrence J. Osteoarthritis and the disc degeneration in an urban population. *Ann Rheum Dis* 1958; **12:** 5–15.
2 Burke M, Fear E, Wright V. Bone and joint changes in pneumatic drillers. *Ann Rheum Dis* 1977; **36:** 276–9.
3 Vincelette P, Laurin C, Levesque H. The footballer's ankle and foot. *Can Med Assoc J* 1972; **107:** 872–7.
4 Klunder K, Rud B, Hansen J. Osteoarthritis of the hip and knee joint in retired football players. *Acta Orth Scand* 1980; **51:** 925–7.

5 Sortland D, Tysvaer A, Storli O. Changes in cervical spine in Association Football. *Br J Sports Med* 1982; **16**: 80–4.

6 Marti B, Knobloch M, Tschopp A, Jucker A, Howald H. Is excessive running predictive of degenerative hip disease? *Br Med J* 1989; **299**: 91–3.

7 Mikkelsen W, Duff I, Dodge H. Age specific prevalence of radiographic abnormalities of the joints of the hands, wrists and cervical spine. *J Chron Dis* 1970; **23**: 151–9.

8 Adams I. Osteoarthritis and sport. *Clin Rheum Dis* 1976; **2**: 523–41.

9 McDermott M, Freyne P. Osteoarthritis in runners with knee pain. *Br J Sports Med* 1983; **17**: 84.

10 Lane N, Bloch D, Jones H, Marshall W, Wood P, Fries J. Long distance running, bone density and osteoarthritis. *JAMA* 1986; **255**: 1147–51.

11 Panush R, Schmidt C, Caldwell J *et al.* Is running associated with degenerative joint disease? *JAMA* 1986; **255**: 1152–4.

12 Puranen J, Ala-Ketola L, Peltokallio P, Saarela J. Running and primary osteoarthritis of the hip. *Br Med J* 1975; **3**: 424–5.

13 Kraus J, D'Ambrosia R, Smith E *et al.* Epidemiological study of severe osteoarthritis. *Orthopaedics* 1978; **1**: 37–42.

14 Balfors B. The course of knee ligament injuries. *Acta Orth Scand* 1982; **53** (suppl 198).

15 Muckle D. Factors affecting the prognosis of meniscectomy in soccer players. *Br J Sports Med* 1983; **17**: 88–90.

16 Gibson T, Davies J, Crane J, Henry A. Knee pain in sports people—a prospective study. *Br J Sports Med* 1987; **21**: 115–17.

17 Doherty M, Watt I, Dieppe P. Localised chondrocalcinosis in post-meniscectomy knees. *Lancet* 1982; **i**: 1207.

18 Fahmy N, Noble J, Williams E. Relationship between meniscal tears and osteoarthritis of the knee. *J Bone Joint Surg* 1981; **63**: 629.

19 Murray B, Duncan C. Athletic activity in adolescence as a factor in degenerative disease of the hip. *J Bone Joint Surg* 1971; **53**: 406–19.

20 Gibson T. Athletic injury clinic. *Demonstration Centre in Rehabilitation Newsletter* 1977; **9**: 6.

21 Editorial. *Br Med J* 1981; **282**: 1014.

22 Robinson A, Darracott J. Chondromalacia patellae. *Ann Phys Med* 1970; **10**: 286–90.

23 Hinnie J, Jankowski J, Brankin E, Sturrock R. Changes in keratan sulphate levels in the serum of a long distance runner. *Br J Rheumatol* 1990; **29**: 314–15.

24 Isdale A, Helliwell P. Athletes and osteoarthritis—is there a relationship? *Br J Rheumatol* 1991; **30**: 67–8.

PART 4
THE LAW AND
LIABILITY

16: Rugby and the Law

EDWARD GRAYSON

IT IS always an honour to be invited to cross the borders from one professional discipline to another, and particularly from the law to medicine. Rumpole's creator, John Mortimer, QC, told the Medico-Legal Society recently that there is a great gap between the medical and legal professions. This surprised me because his father, the late Clifford Mortimer, was also a distinguished barrister, who wrote the leading book on probate law which deals with dead peoples' estates; and he continued in practice after he lost his sight. John Mortimer now is aware of the threads which link the two professions. I have presented him with a copy of *Medicine, Sport and the Law* which begins with my own chapter, Sports Medicine and the Law. This was the first of 15 chapters on sport and the law which I wrote when preparing that publication for the law publishers Butterworths who gave me permission to repeat its contents here and elsewhere.

John Mortimer now realises how sport can bind the two professions, just as it links health and education and the fun element which outside the public and commercial levels is the key to enjoyment of all sport. Rugby football in particular at club, school and student levels is an amateur game, and for health and medical reasons is as important, and, indeed, even more important than what happens at the public level. Since this address was delivered in Bermuda, the *Daily Telegraph* sports column 'Sport Around the World' for Monday 15 July 1991 contained the crucial following paragraphs:

The worst violence in sport occurs on suburban club playing fields, according to a university survey in Australia—and the biggest problems are not restricted to the macho world of rugby league, rugby union, and Aussie rules.

One of the most violent sport is men's lacrosse, and there are also many injuries in men's and women's soccer. Kicking is most commonplace in water polo, and elbowing is a problem in netball.

Almost a third of all players felt the level of violence in their sport, including verbal abuse was excessive, Prof. Ray Vamplew, of Flinders University tells the *Sydney Morning Herald*. And more than half the spectators thought violence was excessive in the sport they were watching.

'One of the worst problems', says Prof. Vamplew, 'is when you get down to the C and D grades, where players said umpires were biased and incompetent. Lots of umpires agreed with that. Professional sport was the best controlled by match officials and this was a key buffer against violence'.

The Law and Liability

At Bermuda I pointed out that one of the most significant names in sport, at both amateur and professional levels, was Corinthian. It gave its name to the Corinthian Football Club which amalgamated with the Casuals to become the present Corinthian–Casuals Football Club.

When I was a very young barrister I used to receive instructions from a solicitor who had played for both clubs, and had an amateur approach to my professional fees. When I told him that I thought he was more Casual than Corinthian in his obligations at that level he decided that he would experiment with his credit practices elsewhere. Correspondingly, when I first drew attention to the criminal element in sporting violence I also found myself unpopular with certain elements in the sporting establishment who falsely claimed that sport could look after itself without any outside intervention from lawyers. Any uncertainties which this undoubted hostility created were finally dispelled by two landmark contributions in the *British Medical Journal* on 23 December 1978. J.E. Davies, then Research Registrar, and T. Gibson, Consultant Physician, recorded in an article entitled 'Injuries in Rugby Union Football' based upon their experiences at Guy's Hospital Injuries Athletics Clinic:

In a prospective study of 185 players attached to 10 British rugby clubs . . . foul play might have caused as many as 47 (31%) of all reported injuries. Complete eradication of deliberately dangerous play would considerably reduce the high incidence of injuries in this sport.

On different pages J.P.R. Williams, Surgical Registrar, and Professor B. McKibbin, in the Department of Traumatic and Orthopaedic Surgery at Cardiff Royal Infirmary, warned in an article entitled 'Cervical Spine Injuries in Rugby Union Football':

Referees and coaches should be aware of the dangers of scrum collapses, especially as it seems to be an increasingly popular tactic to bring about this purposefully.

Not only did this crucial medical evidence from such impeccable sporting medical sources corroborate my own conclusions based on what I had witnessed with my own eyes for too long in the preceding years. They also corroborated the conclusions of unacknowledged criminality identified in the 1966 World Soccer Cup competition which the principal victim, the Brazilian star, Pelé, chronicled in 1977, in *My Life and the Beautiful Game* written with Robert L. Fish (at pp. 144–5):

. . . against Bulgaria . . . I had been the target of merciless attacks from Zechev of Bulgaria throughout the entire game. Zechev did everything he could physically to cripple me, and the referee, Jim Finney, gave neither me nor any of the others on our team the protection we had a right to expect from an official in a game . . .

Morais, of Portugal, had a field day fouling me, eventually putting me out of the

[94]

game. He tripped me, and when I was stumbling to the ground he leaped at me, feet first, and cut me down completely. It wasn't until I actually saw the films of the game that I realised what a terribly vicious double-foul it was. The stands came to their feet screaming at the foul, but the English referee, George McCabe, allowed Morais to remain on the field, although again, even in the most inexperienced league in the world, he would have been thrown out for either of the two fouls, let alone both. Dr Gosling and Mario Americo came to help me from the field, and Brazil went on to play with ten men and ended up eliminated from the tournament.

Those impressions of what the films showed for Pelé have been confirmed by my own viewing at least seven times of the nationally marketed official film of the 1966 World Cup Competition, *Goal* by its scriptwriter and the *Sunday Times* football correspondent, Brian Glanville, and also *The Times'* senior sportswriter, David Miller. The consequences legally are independently and interdependently sixfold as set out below. They were all repeated 14 years later during the semi-final of the 1982 World Cup competition in Spain. The West German goalkeeper Schumacher assaulted the French defender Battiston in a manner condemned internationally by the sporting press. Yet as David Miller recorded in his book on the 1966 World Cup, *The Boys of '66: England's Lost Glory* at p. 21:

Any dignified sport would have suspended for life the West German goalkeeper for his atrocious foul in the 1982 semi-final, which shamefully handicapped the French. From FIFA there was no more than a murmur.

Battiston's 1982 West German experience and Pelé's Portuguese and Bulgarian experiences in the 1966 World Cup created a classic combination of circumstances which *could* and *should* have demonstrated—but did not—how all six legal layers acted upon and with each other in an effective policy because the fouls merited the following sanctions action:

1 *Playing* sending off from field punishment;

2 *Playing penal* in breach of Law 12—violent conduct or serious foul play;

3 *Administrative* suspension or dismissal from competition in the manner suffered 12 years later by Scotland's star winger sent home from the 1978 World Cup in Argentina following a positive drugs test in breach of FIFA rules but lawfully prescribed under Parliament's Misuse of Drugs Act 1971 (see Chapter 11, *Sport and the Law*, Butterworths, 1988: 235);

4 *National* prosecution under Section 47 of the Offences Against the Person Act, 1861, for assault occasioning actual bodily harm;

5 *International governing body* as in (2) above with censure upon referees and FIFA noted by David Miller for abdicating responsibilities; and

6 *Overseas national* as in (3) above, with the precedents from other violent visitors or criminal offenders to UK shores.

The rugby scene: 1977 onwards

Although these experiences cited above related to the round ball rather than the oval-shaped version, the medico–legal relationship is the same for both games; and the year of Pelé's accusations, which can never be challenged, had a double significance for rugby union football. The Scottish international referee Norman Sanson sent off Geoff Wheel and Willie Duggan for punching each other in the Wales v. Ireland international match at Cardiff; and a broken jaw in two places from an off-the-ball tackle ended a year later with the first ever traceable criminal prosecution for foul play on the rugby field *(R. v. Billinghurst* [1978] Crim. Law Rev. 553).

Coincidentally and ironically the trial took place precisely 100 years after the criteria for criminal foul play had been established in 1878 following a prosecution for a soccer fatality. They were reaffirmed 20 years later in another fatal soccer death trial, and consolidated generally as recently as 1975. How I explained the position in Butterworth's *Sport and the Law* published in 1988 at pp. 130–1 appears as follows.

In *Bradshaw's Case* ([1878] 14, Cox CC 83), a jury acquitted a footballer in a friendly game on a manslaughter charge after evidence had been given from one of the two umpires then in charge of the game that no unfair play occurred. During prosecuting counsel's opening speech to the jury, Bramwell LJ interrupted a reference to the game's rules to say (p. 48):

whether within the rules or not, the prisoner would be guilty of manslaughter if while committing an unlawful act he caused the death of the deceased.

His summing-up (at p. 85) to the jury included these words:

If a man is playing according to the rules and practice of the game and not going beyond it, it may be reasonable to infer that he is not actuated by any malicious motive or intention, and that he is not acting in a manner which he knows will be likely to be productive of death or injury. But, independent of the rules, if the prisoner intended to cause serious hurt to the deceased, or if he knew that, in charging as he did, he might produce serious injury and was indifferent and reckless as to whether he would produce serious injury or not, then the act would be unlawful. In either case he would be guilty of a criminal act and you must find him guilty; if you are of a contrary opinion you will acquit him.

On the evidence the jury returned a verdict of Not Guilty.

Twenty years later in *Moore's case* ([1898] 14 TLR 229) the evidence was that the accused jumped with his knees against the victim's back. This threw him violently against a knee of the goalkeeper, causing an internal rupture and ultimate death, a few days afterwards. He, too, was charged with manslaughter; and on this occasion the verdict was Guilty.

Hawkins J's summing-up to the jury explained (pp. 229–30):

the rules of the game were quite immaterial . . . it did not matter whether the prisoner broke the rules or not. Football was a lawful game, but it was a rough one and persons who played it must be careful to restrain themselves so as not to do bodily harm to any other person. No one had a right to use force which was likely to injure another, and if he did use such force and death resulted, the crime of manslaughter had been committed.
. . . If a blow were struck recklessly which caused a man to fall, and if in falling he struck against something and was injured and died, the person who struck the blow was guilty of manslaughter, even though the blow itself would not have caused injury.

Nearly a century after *Bradshaw's case* in *R. v. Venna* ([1975] 3 All ER 788), a more recent Court of Appeal dismissed appeals against convictions for assault occasioning actual bodily harm and Public Order offences in a non-sporting context. The reserved judgment after two days of legal argument included the following significant sentence (at p. 793 f–g):

R. v. Bradshaw [1878] 14 Cox CC 85 can be read as supporting the view that unlawful physical force applied recklessly constitutes a criminal assault.

What constitutes 'recklessly' has been the subject of such subsequent gymnastics by the higher judiciary in the House of Lords that they moved the learned Editors of the leading practitioners' 'bible' in the criminal courts, *Archbold*, in the Preface to the 41st edition, at page v, to describe them as 'a challenge even to the most gifted of Her Majesty's trial judges'. 'Wildly impulsive' is the definition in *The Oxford Minidictionary*. Disregarding the consequences is the yardstick used by practitioners. For present purposes it would be advisable for each citation from Bramwell LJ, Hawkins J and the Court of Appeal in *Venna* to be hung alongside Lord Hanworth's words in *Doyle's case*.

That cross-reference to *Doyle's Case* was to the classic comment of one of Lord Denning's predecessors as Master of the Rolls when the famous Irish heavyweight boxer Jack Doyle sued unsuccessfully in the Court of Appeal for his forfeited purse after he had been disqualified for foul fighting against the future President of the British Boxing Board of Control, Jack Petersen, for heavyweight championship of Great Britain in 1933. Rejecting Doyle's claim, Lord Hanworth explained,

It is as much in the interests of the plaintiff himself as of any other contestant that there should be rules for clean fighting and that he should be protected against his adversary's misconduct in hitting below the belt or doing anything of the sort.

(*Doyle v. White City Stadium Ltd* [1935] 1kB 110.)

Consenting to lawful sporting injuries

Boxing more than any competitive sport illuminates the universal misconception about consenting to sporting injury, i.e. *volens*, voluntary acceptance. A participant accepts the normal lawful risks so that *volenti non fit injuria:* i.e. that to which someone consents cannot be considered an actionable injury. No civilised legal system would ever countenance and apply this principle to unlawful, unsporting, misconduct.

Erroneously in the *Billinghurst case* the defence was argued of the victim having consented to the broken jaw suffered from an off-the-ball tackle. Because that case was the first ever traceable trial for a rugby injury the conviction in 1978 resulted in a suspended sentence of 9 months. Resulting from a progressive failure since then, of the clubs and governing bodies to curtail the growing violence on the field in the manner evidenced by Davies and Gibson in the *British Medical Journal* on 23 December 1988, and the *Daily Telegraph*'s 'Sport Around the World' on Monday 15 July 1991, the courts had gradually responded with a progressive scale of *immediate* as distinct from *suspended* custodial sentences. Thus 10 years onwards *The Times* for 15 September 1988 recorded the current tariff which now stands at 18 months imprisonment for a broken cheekbone caused by an amateur rugby player in a club match kicking an opponent during the course of play (*R. v. Lloyd*: Bristol Crown Court).

By contrast to such undoubted criminality, my own broken fibula from a mistimed tackle during the Oxford University soccer trials, when I stabbed the ground instead of the ball which had already been whisked away from my reach, is a classic example of the *volens* principle. The subsequent mistreatment was equally a classic example of medical negligence, which my parents did not pursue as I would certainly do if I would have suffered from that cause today.

Negligence as well as trespass to the person creating the claim for civil assault have each been activated for damage awards for violent foul football play. Unknown to all of us in Bermuda, the Australian Courts were considering a claim by an international Australian professional rugby league player, Steve Rogers, for a broken jaw caused by a head-high tackle from an opponent Mark Bugden, which was outside the laws of the game. He succeeded in recovering $68 000 against not only the offender but also the employer club, Canterbury Bankstown, on the principle of vicarious liability for assault, judgment being delivered in the New South Wales Common Law Court on 14 December 1990.

That injury occurred during 1985, the year in which the English Court of Appeal upheld a county court award of £4000 for a broken leg caused by a foul slide tackle in a local league soccer match, on the basis of a negligence claim, i.e. based on a 'reckless disregard of the plaintiff's safety which fell far below the standards which might reasonably be expected in anyone pursuing the game' (*Condon v. Basi* [1988] 2 All ER 453). The Court of Appeal also proclaimed that a higher duty lies upon a First Division player than one at a lower level, inevitably because of the greater skilled player's capacity to exercise greater care to avoid injury.

Medical sporting negligence

The criteria operated in *Condon v. Basi* (supra) will be recognised by the medical profession as analogous to the classic criteria laid down by McNair J in *Bolam v. Friern Hospital Management Committee* [1957] 2 All ER 118,

as a rule a doctor is not negligent if he acts in accordance with a practice accepted at the time as proper by a responsible body of medical opinion even though other doctors adopt a different practice. In short, the law imposes a duty of care, but the standard of care is a matter of medical judgment.

United Kingdom conventional sporting traditions in the past of not involving the law with sport have doubtless contributed to an absence of precedents at this level. Two Canadian cases illustrate the dangers if doctors ignore the standards expected of them. One was from British Columbia and the other from Ontario.

A direct example of liability was established by the Ontario Court of Appeal. A 41-year-old tool and dye worker broke his right ankle when playing soccer with his son. A negligently erroneous X-ray prescription requiring attention to the right foot was compounded by a cascade of consequential errors involving several medical practitioners, including a radiologist, all of whom consolidated the earlier misdiagnosis. This resulted in the appellate court's confirmation of the trial judge's ruling that 'One negligent doctor could be liable for the additional loss caused by the other.' The appeal court also upheld the damages award of $50 000 for general damages, which included $34 465 for loss of income up to the date of trial (*Price v. Milawski* [1978] 82 DLR (3d) 130).

For vicarious liability upon a sporting organisation because of medical negligence, the British Columbia Court of Appeal upheld the trial judge on a claim by a 28-year-old Canadian professional ice-hockey player, Mike Robitaille, against his former employer hockey club, Vancouver, known as the 'Canucks' (see *Robitaille v. Vancouver Hockey Club Ltd* [1981] DLR (3rd) 288).

Sustained complaints to various club officials and doctors of developing injuries suffered in play were rejected in what were found judicially to be arrogant and high-handed forms of conduct. The neglect proved resulted in considerable personal and professional losses and suffering. The doctors' nexus with the club to establish vicarious liability comprised a relatively modest bonus of $2500, season tickets, free parking and access to the club lounge. The appeal court upheld the trial judge's evidential findings that

the measure of control asserted by the defendant over the doctors in carrying out their work was substantial. The degree of control need not be complete in order to establish vicarious liability. In the case of a professional person, the absence of control and direction over the manner of doing the work is of little significance: *Morren v. Swinton and Pendelbury Borough Council* [1965] 2 All ER 349, 351.

Also confirmed were the trial judge's damages awards of:
1 $175 000 for loss of professional hockey income;
2 $85 000 for loss of future income other than from professional hockey; and
3 $40 000 for the traditional pain, suffering and loss of enjoyment of life.
Of equal significance for all sportspersons was a concurrent approval of the appeal court of the trial judge's conclusion about the plaintiff's contributory negligence. He was held to be

20% at fault because of his failure to take any action [i.e. to complain] to protect his own interest was less than reasonable. There was evidence upon which Esson J could find that Robitaille was negligent . . . the trial judge correctly distinguished cases . . . which dealt with factory workers . . . dealing here with a highly paid experienced modern day professional athlete and not a factory worker responding to the mores of olden times.

The plaintiff's contributory negligence assessment by the Court of not pursuing his medical complaints to agencies outside the negligent club's control earlier than he did was possibly harsh. Nevertheless, the trial judge heard extensive oral evidence, and his final awards which included aggravated and exemplary damages demonstrated his ultimate awareness of the plaintiff's overriding and justifiable grievance for medical neglect which created a clearcut vicarious liability.

The reverse side of this particular coin will be the doctor who allows himself or herself to be persuaded by an athlete, coach, director or management to participate in any activity or competition, or when any participant is by an ordinary medical criteria unfit or not sufficiently fit, without risk of exacerbating a pre-existing medical condition. The former Southampton and England footballer, Mike Channon, who now trains racehorses, commented after one of his mounts won a classic race notwithstanding a built-in corn condition, that out of 800 soccer matches in which he had played, 100% fitness had not existed in at least 100 of them. He did not explain whether or not he had made this disclosure to his club's medical advisers.

Significantly, another international footballer, Andy Gray who became the only recipient ever of both the Player of the Year and Young Player of the Year awards in the same season from the Professional Footballers Association, wrote during 1986 in *Shades of Gray* at p. 96:

It's often said in dressing rooms that horses have better treatment than humans, and it's true as far as some football clubs go . . . Happily, most clubs, especially first and second division sides, have tightened up on their medical care in recent seasons. But I could still name you a team of class players whose careers have been finished early because they were abused so badly.

Conclusion

How far that judgment applies to rugby football, each club and each medical adviser must judge for himself or herself. Certainly the sporting–leisure explosion with greater longevity and unemployment alongside a technological–mechanical revolution in international society means that the need for sporting–medical services will never diminish. Furthermore, as violence in society shows no signs of diminishing, and sport will always mirror and reflect the widest social spectrum, it is as well for all concerned with the welfare of rugby football to remember the experience of John Davies and Terry Gibson (cited on p. 94 above) in relation to the wider conclusions of *Glaister's Medical Jurisprudence and Toxicology* (13th edition, 1973, p. 256, end of chapter headed 'The Medico–legal Aspects of Wounds'):

the examiner should direct his attention to the reconstruction of the cause of the injuries. He should first decide the instrument, then the degree of violence, the possibility of accident, the direction of the wound, and the relative position of the parties.

For sporting injuries caused by violent foul play this formula cannot be improved. It also can be seen as a corollary to what appears to have been the secret for the professional success of the first Lord Horder in his early days at Bart's at the turn of the century before his new legendary but deserved eminence. This was explained by his son's memoir, *The Little Genius* (1966) as,

that preoccupation with the postmortem room . . . and an examination of the body after death was often, as it sometimes still is, the only way to arrive at the truth about a particular case, to confirm or upset a diagnosis, and to push forward the frontiers of knowledge in general. There is no arguing with the corpse on the slab.

If rugby, soccer, and all mobile body contact sports are to be saved from self-destruction and ending as corpses on a social slab the administrators, now obsessed with commercial and sponsorship services, must heed the messages which the medico–legal professions in harmony together on the evidence outlined here can alone provide. Without that harmony, sport as a vehicle for health and enjoyment cannot survive.

Discussion

ENGLAND: In 1976 I had a scholarship to the Kan Hospital in Basle where I spent 3 months in Switzerland and joined the Basle rugby club. The scenario is an international one and I would like to ask a question as I was appointed honorary doctor to Basle rugby club at the time: we trained twice a week in Germany; we played once a week somewhere in Switzerland; and occasionally in mid-week we played in France. Who sues me, how and why?

GRAYSON: I am glad you have raised that question. I am still trying to find out that when a British doctor goes overseas, does he have to register with the overseas country where he is in occupation in order to be in a position to carry out medical advice or treatment, because as I understand it, if he does not get himself registered, even temporarily with the overseas country he may be in breach of some medical statute.

PAYNE: For the purpose of practising medicine you are subject to the medical act in the UK, and the medical act provides for the doctor to practice medicine. In other words to practice medicine you do not have to be registered in the UK. The situation is the same in other countries in that you have to be registered, to hold yourself out to be a practitioner, but you do not have to be registered or even qualified to actually practice medicine, if someone will let you practice medicine.

GRAYSON: So British Medical Qualification is a passport to practice medicine all over the world?

PAYNE: You do not have to be qualified at all. What you cannot do, presumably it would be in a breach of various medical acts around the world, is to hold yourself out to be a doctor.

GRAYSON: Mr England, in his travels, therefore, would be subject to the laws of negligence or criminal liability if anything were to go wrong, just as an overseas doctor of any sport teaching in the UK would be called upon in an emergency to practice upon a British player and has failed in his medico–legal liability.

PAYNE: Likewise, you do not have to be qualified to prescribe medicines as long as they are not controlled drugs or prescription-only.

DAVIES: Before we close this morning, as this is a fairly global conference, I would like a bit of input from people in the other countries. Have you had any liability problems? Dr Keno, has any player in Japan now been convicted of assault?

KENO: Yes.

DAVIES: Fiji? No? France? No?

PENE: I do not think so.

GRAYSON: There was a prosecution in France—an English player who went out to France—who may have been acquitted. Civilised countries throughout the world, thank goodness, have a common denominator with various statutory qualifications that if a chap commits violence on a playing field then the same clinical liability arises throughout the world.

DAVIES: What about liability in South Africa?

HUGO: Not yet—we have warned them and I think it has been discussed on many levels, and we are looking forward to what is happening in Britain and elsewhere.

CHASE: What is the doctors responsibility or liability when treating a patient and then telling the coach that he is not fit to play?

GRAYSON: Your relationship is to the patient, even if you are under contract to the club. There seems to be a loose area which is why the Vancouver case was important because there was no contract but there was control. My reading of the law is, and there may be some disagreement, that the overriding duty of the doctor must be to the patient, and if in fact the coach insists on the patient playing, the doctor says that he plays against my advice. When I told this to the Football Association meeting and suggested that it must go into writing, the chairman of the FA said that it was the best advice I could ever give.

17: The Medico–Legal Hazards of Rugby Football

SIMON D.W.PAYNE

THE SPORTS physician may be surprised to find that the application of law has an important role in sports medicine. Furthermore the normative medical values of physicians who provide their services to sportsmen and women, when combined with principles of law and ethics can, by synthesis of these two elements, produce a third element which may be characterized as an exercise in preventive medicine. It is important that doctors

Table 17.1 Responsibilities of the doctor engaged in treating sportsmen

Code	Purpose	Sanction
Criminal law	Protection of society against undesirable activities	Fine or prison
Civil law	Protection of society against poor standards (competence)	'Damages' paid in compensation
Ethical considerations	Maintenance of professional integrity (conduct)	Deregistration (GMC)

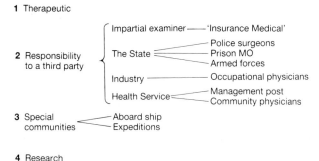

Fig. 17.1 The doctor–patient relationships which may apply to a doctor treating sportsmen.

understand their responsibilities in both civil and criminal matters, and are also sensitive to the ethical pitfalls that exist for the unwary (Table 17.1). With regard to pitfalls of litigation the tort of negligence which traditionally has been perceived as having no application in sports medicine has produced a number of important reported cases where doctors providing their services to sportsmen have been found legally liable (q.v.). Furthermore, the issue may be complicated by the fact that the doctor–patient relationship can be significantly altered in sports medicine. Most doctors who provide their services in sports medicine do so on an honorary basis. Although there are a small number of dedicated sports physicians, in practice most are derived from the ranks of general practitioners or orthopaedic surgeons.

In considering the doctor–patient relationship with respect to sports medicine it is helpful to consider first the types of relationship that can potentially exist. There are at least four types (Fig. 17.1). The first and most commonly encountered is described as the 'therapeutic relationship'. Here the doctor acts only in the best medical interests of his or her patient and exercises the fundamental principles of medical philosophy and practice for the benefit of the patient, to save life, to promote healing and to alleviate suffering. The application of these principles may be characterised as an exhibition of beneficence. Arising from the therapeutic doctor–patient relationship there are implications in issues of consent and confidentiality. In a therapeutic relationship the doctor is prohibited by the ethical code from disclosing secrets learnt about the patient unless the patient's consent is forthcoming. In other types of doctor–patient relationship there may be a responsibility to a third party, for example in the case of a medical examination for insurance purposes. Here the doctor will pass on to the insurance company information, which, under normal circumstances, is secret and which the patient generally may not wish others to know. The doctor's position in this ethical matter is protected by virtue of the fact that the doctor always has (or should have) the patient's express consent to pass on that information.

Similarly, doctors who work in various capacities for the state are called on from time to time to perform acts which cannot be construed as being beneficial to the patient. In the days of capital punishment, a prison doctor would be present to confirm death at judicial hanging, a function which cannot in any way be described as being in the patient's interest.

Furthermore, in industry and other non-clinical branches of the health service, doctors may provide information to other parties which in normal situations the patient may not wish them to do. A further example of modified doctor–patient relationship is seen in isolated communities, for example aboard ship and on expeditions to remote parts. The beneficence that a doctor would normally show towards an individual patient has to be taken in context with the viability of the expedition itself when the welfare of the party as a whole may conflict with the interests of an individual. Here the principles that would normally apply to alleviate suffering, promote health and save life might not be expressed on a one to one basis as they would be in a normal therapeutic relationship.

In research, on a philosophical level, no direct benefit will necessarily accrue to the individual patient as a direct result of the trial or experiment undertaken, other than through the benefit to society in general that may obtain through the advance in medical knowledge produced.

As a separate parameter in the doctor–patient relationship one should consider the varieties of attitude which the patient may exhibit with respect to autonomy. It is possible for the relationship at one extreme to be completely paternalistic and at the other for the control with regard to treatment and investigation to be devolved to the patient (Fig. 17.2). In

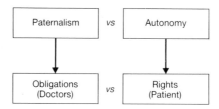

Fig. 17.2 Attitudes which may influence doctor–patient relationships.

British medicine a somewhat paternalistic attitude tends to be seen. Broadly speaking, patients seem happy to abdicate responsibility for medical decision making to their doctors, perhaps because they do not particularly want to know the details of their investigation and treatment. This attitude, which tends to be more prevalent in older generations of patients, does however place upon the doctor a greater responsibility with regard to the standard of care provided, thus causing the doctor also to adopt a more cautious approach to investigation and treatment in the best interests of the patient.

This traditional approach should be contrasted with an alternative attitude which is emerging in which the patient demands greater autonomy over the medical decision making process that takes place, producing a subtle change in the doctor–patient dynamic in which the patient defines an expectation with regard to the standard of care to be delivered in terms of 'rights to a level of quality'. This may be viewed as the counterpart of the duty of care of the doctor which is a more prominent feature within the framework civil law coloured by paternalistic attitudes. In consideration of attitudes with respect to delivery of health care the autonomous and paternalistic approaches may be thought of as being at opposite ends of the same spectrum. It seems probable that in a population of younger individuals, where sporting activity may be more prevalent, patients are more likely to wish to exert greater control over their own destiny in the investigation and treatment of conditions from which they suffer. Such a desire for greater autonomy may have its expression in a requirement for more detailed information about the investigation or treatment which the doctor is planning to provide.

The sports physician is therefore likely to be confronted relatively frequently with patients who demand greater autonomy with regard to treatment decisions and furthermore is quite likely to be providing a service where the doctor may have a responsibility to a third party, such as a governing body or team management. It is likely that there will be a strict therapeutic relationship between the doctor and the patient but that the relationship would be more akin to the type of doctor–patient interaction seen in occupational medicine. This is important because there are significant practical implications associated with the different types of doctor–patient relationship that may be seen. Normally, in a therapeutic relationship, there would be free and frank exchange of clinical information, possibly including details of a personal nature, between the patient's GP and any specialist to whom the patient was referred, where both practitioners are acting in a therapeutic sense. Generally, there would be no need to obtain the patient's consent for such information to be transferred (although the patient's wish to prohibit such an exchange should usually be respected). Contrast this with the situation where the doctor has a responsibility to a third party—such as a 'company doctor' where the interests of the company have to be taken into account alongside those of the patient. Here the patient's express consent for disclosure is required. When a specialist considers the initiation of treatment for a patient, the GP's consent is not required where the relationship is of a therapeutic type, but consent from the GP should be sought before initiating treatment if the patient is seeing a doctor who is fulfilling the role of an occupational physician. Again this is because the function of the occupational physician is to provide advice to the organisation for which he or she works. This may involve determining a patient's fitness to work and whether or not any restrictions on the patient should be placed.

Assuming therefore that the sports physician sometimes functions in circumstances where he or she may not bear a normal therapeutic relationship with the patient and furthermore that the doctor may be involved with patients who seek to exert greater autonomy over their destiny, consider the position of the team doctor who is approached by team management for medical information about a player which may affect team selection where that player has asked specifically for that information to remain confidential. Clearly the doctor has an ethical dilemma, for to breach confidence by fully informing management of the complete nature of the player's condition could, on a theoretical basis at least, lead to censure from the doctors' disciplinary body (the General Medical Council) whereas to fail to disclose could possibly lead to economic loss arising from the poor performance of a key player for which the club could hold the doctor responsible if the facts became known. This potential problem could be eased if the relationship between the doctor and team management were to become more formalised. The doctor and the patient would then be more clearly aware of the nature of the relationship that existed between them and commercial embarrassment between the doctor and the club would be avoided.

A definition of sport is difficult to find. The *Concise Oxford Dictionary* indicates that it is an activity in which enjoyment is an integral part. One of the best definitions has been coined by UNESCO: 'a physical activity which has the character of play and involves a struggle with oneself or with others in a confrontation of natural elements'. This is nevertheless an incomplete picture. Sport certainly involves exertion which is usually physical, although an intellectual game such as chess may be considered by many to be sport in which case the definition of 'exertion' ought perhaps to be widened to include physical or mental activity. Exertion nevertheless must be an integral part of the definition of sport in the same way that competition is also an element. A further factor which it is important to acknowledge is that there must be an acceptance of a framework of rules. Such rules exist on playing, organisation and national levels (Table 17.2). The regulations governing the shape of the pitch, the size of the ball, the number of players per team and the rules of play, both facilitative and restrictive, are all examples of playing rules. The administrative rules concerning the way in which the game is organised and set up within a given union are also well known. However, many do not realise that activities seen within the game, involving players, advisers and professionals, are also subject to national rules through legislation and the common law. Criminal law records a number of cases in which violent foul play has been a feature (Table 17.3). In each case a clear breach of playing and administrative rules has occurred which unfortunately were not dealt with effectively at these levels. The resulting unresolved grievances have therefore produced prosecutions for criminal assault, resulting in conviction in a number of cases, some with custodial sentences. In civil law the high watermark of litigation between players on the pitch occurred in

Table 17.2 Rules as they may apply at different levels of organisation

Playing rules
Descriptive/facilitative
Restrictive/penal

Administrative rules
Organisational
Maintenance of standards and safety
Disciplinary

National rules
Civil law
Criminal law

Table 17.3 Breach of the rules and of the criminal law (*R. v. Bishop* [1986] *The Times* 12 October 1986)

1985: Punched opponent in club match: concussion
Playing rules—not seen by referee
Administrative rules—ignored by club officials
National 'rules': Prosecution for criminal assault
   Conviction
    1 month imprisonment (reduced to suspended sentence by Court of Appeal)

Condon v. Basi (Table 17.4). Here, during an amateur soccer match, a tackle in which a leg fracture was sustained was considered to be so gross a foul tackle by those who witnessed it that a successful suit in negligence and trespass was brought and damages of some £4000 were paid.

Doctors who have traditionally thought themselves immune from civil litigation when providing their services in a sports context may wish to consider the salutary case of *Robitaille v. The Vancouver Ice Hockey Company Ltd* (Table 17.5). Mike Robitaille was a professional ice hockey player whose repeated complaints of injury were ignored by the club doctor. He sustained damage which curtailed his playing career and the doctor and the club were found negligent. The club was adjudged vicariously liable for the doctor's negligence and this was perhaps fortunate for the doctor because otherwise

Table 17.4 Application of civil law (*Condon v. Basi* [1985] 2 AER 453)

Foul tackle during amateur soccer match: broken leg
Claim in negligence and trespass
£4000 damages awarded (affirmed in Court of Appeal)

Table 17.5 Civil litigation in sport—an example (*Robitaille v. Vancouver Ice Hockey Club Ltd* [1981] 3 DLR 288)

Professional ice hockey player: repeated complaints of injury
Club doctor (no contract) provides incomplete examination and no effective treatment
   Neck damage not diagnosed
   Playing career shortened
Doctor and club found negligent (club vicariously liable)

Award: $175 000 for loss of professional hockey income
       $85 000 for future loss of other income
       $50 000 for pain, suffering and loss of amenity

Total: $310 000

---

he could have been made personally liable. An award of over a third of a million dollars in damages was made in 1981, upheld on appeal. This result exemplifies how civil liability is an important issue for doctors providing their services to sports people and doctors so affected are usually personally liable.

Civil liability is a risk for all professional practice. A confusion may arise because the dictionary provides an English linguistic understanding of the word negligence which is significantly different from the legal definition. This is strictly defined as 'a breach of duty of care resulting in damage'. There are thus three elements: (a) a duty of care between the doctor and his patient; (b) a breach of that duty; and (c) loss or damage. The law of negligence exists to provide compensation for loss which may include pain, suffering, loss of amenity and economic loss. The common law and its system of precedent will determine fairly consistently the monetary value which may be associated with pain, suffering and loss of amenity of various kinds. Economic loss however is very variable and depends on such things as earning capacity of the individual and the extent to which this has been compromised, and the number of productive years the individual could have expected to have enjoyed had these not been curtailed by the act of negligence. The professional responsibilities or the duty of care which the sports physician owes to his or her patient should be recognised wherever a sporting injury requires treatment, a breach of that duty alongside a reasonably foreseeable risk of injury creates a liability in negligence. The standard of care required is determined under English law by the case of *Bolam v. Friern Barnet Health Authority*, a landmark case in medical negligence. This is defined as the standard of 'the ordinary skilled man exercising and professing to have that special skill: a man need not possess the highest expert skill. It is sufficient if he exercises the ordinary skill of an ordinary competent man exercising that particular art'. Doctors providing services in sports medicine are therefore required to display the skill of the average sports physician. The fact that the average standard of such practitioners is increasing through education means that a doctor must achieve a level of competence which is significantly higher than that of even a few years ago. Litigation in medical practice generally is on the increase on both sides of the Atlantic. The Canadian Medical Protective Association's analysis of their legal action per 1000 members indicates an approximate 10-fold rise from 1960 to 1986. In the USA, malpractice settlements are also increasing and by 1985 the average litigation settlement for medical malpractice had exceeded $1 million. There are a number of reasons for these massive numbers seen in North America, not least of which is the use of the contingency system. This means that the lawyer running the case is paid nothing if the case is lost but receives a substantial payment if the case is won, up to 50% in some incidences. It is however felt that this system provides a greater accessibility to the law for the general public, as contrasted with the system seen in the UK where one's legal fees to solicitors and barristers are payable whether the case is won or lost. A further important difference between the USA and UK systems is that in the USA malpractice cases are tried by jury, who also may determine the quantum of damages. In the UK similar cases are heard by a high court judge sitting alone.

Table 17.6 Summary of adopted recommendations of the Medical Advisory Committee of the IRFB (1978) for preventive medicine in sport

Elimination of high tackle
Scrummaging law changes
Reduce impact
Prevent collapse
Prevent scrum rotation
Maul *vs.* ruck
Encourage players to stay on feet
Encourage quick release after tackle
Drugs/doping
No injectable analgesics
Player size (schools)
Avoid mismatch
Mouthguards
Concluson
3-week ban

It is important to remember that for doctors who are touring abroad, medical services provided therein are subject to the local jurisdiction and a touting doctor could therefore be sued within these courts. It is essential therefore that any doctor accompanying a visiting team who contemplates undertaking any medical procedure of whatever description is adequately covered by insurance. This may be a particular problem for the USA and Canada where the UK protection organisations do not write business.

Doctors who associate themselves with sports medicines have a duty not only to treat patients who appear with injuries, but also to endeavour to reduce the incidence of injury by collecting and analysing information in order that patterns of damage may be identified.

The American Association of Neurologists has produced striking improvements in the nature and extent of injuries occurring to American professional football players following a study taking place between 1968 and 1973. This led to modifications of laws, equipment and coaching techniques and illustrates what can be done if the full force of medical evidence is presented to governing bodies in a way which cannot be ignored. Likewise the Medical Committee of the IRFB have made certain recommendations with respect to playing and administrative rules which have brought about a reduction in certain injuries (Table 17.6).

Discussion

DAVIES: The standard of skill required by law makes it all the more important that we form an association of rugby medicine doctors. If we do that, perhaps we could also in conjunction with the Royal College of Physicians produce a diploma of sports medicine. I think these are very important points from a medico–legal point of view.

JONES: The one thing that worries me—Swansea play an occasional game of rugby against Llanelli and Neath, and after the game there are usually quite a few with bumps and bruises. One tends to give, say, ibuprofen. What of those who may have had asthma in the past or a duodenal ulcer? Let us say that within the next few hours an NSAID provokes an acute asthmatic attack or gastrointestinal bleeding? Where do we stand? Should we give these drugs or not?

PAYNE: There are two aspects I think. First of all, the ethical aspect which is the fact that you are not the patient's GP. Theoretically speaking you should not really be treating them, and if you are going to treat them it should be with the consent of the GP and you should keep the GP informed. It sounds a bit cumbersome but this is what should happen.

The aspect which is perhaps more important is that of civil liability. Once you have given your advice, even if it is informal advice, you set up a legal liability. If the standard of this advice is below that of the average practitioner and the patient suffers as a result then you are liable in negligence and damages are payable. There are two things you must do. First of all you must be circumspect about treating patients in the circumstances you describe, especially if you do not know the past medical history and if you are using agents with significant side effects. I am sure that you may be subject to a degree of pressure and coercion by players. If you do not know the player at all I think it would be very unwise to offer them treatment. Secondly it is important that you have adequate skills in relation to the field in which you practice. Sports medicine and perhaps even rugby medicine are specialisms if not specialities in their own right.

BOTTOMLEY: There are plenty of precedents for treating patients in an emergency without the consent of a GP—particularly for visiting players where it is clearly impossible to get the consent of the patient's GP. Would we be covering ourselves rather better if we made a point of writing a note to the patient's doctor and asking the patient, under clear instruction, to take that letter to the doctor, detailing the treatment that was given?

PAYNE: Quite frankly, you should be doing that anyway. Yes.

CHASE: I just wanted to say that from my own experience I think that you are probably covered for the majority of the liability that you face in the USA—at least if you do have the informed consent of the patient—and you tell him what the drug is that you are giving him and you ask him if he has asthma, for instance, or a history of gastrointestinal problems.

The next point would be to have somebody sign a waiver that they had been informed of this medication and the risks. Everyone should cover themselves as they feel comfortable, but I agree with you—have insurance. You ought not to be doing this without insurance. Remember there are a lot of people who will come out to take care of a team that are not sports doctors. They are going to be held to the standard of a person who knows how to treat sports injuries.

McLATCHIE: With the onset of this year in the UK there is something which is called crown indemnity which has been brought in, which means that a surgeon working for the health authority is covered for negligence claims within the hospital itself. Our Medical Defence Union—and I am with the Scottish one—wrote to us offering a reduction on our annual fee but covering non-paid items like sports medicine. Does that cover our civil liability then?

PAYNE: Yes, providing that the agreement that you have with your protection organisation includes an indemnity benefit then you should be covered. It should be stressed however that the organisations which provide such cover in the UK (the Medical Protection Society, Medical Defence Union and the Medical and Dental Defence Union of Scotland) all now have different subscription policies—some of which, like the MPS, are based on perceived risk of the practitioners and others of which are based on declared income. Superimposed on these different systems there are various categories of membership, some of which have no indemnity benefit. Under these circumstances you may not be covered. If you are unsure of your category of membership you should check with your protection organisation.

MORGAN: Can I ask a Welsh side touring in Canada not to prosecute through the American courts and sign a disclaimer to that effect?

PAYNE: You cannot contract out of liability. Such a disclaimer would be likely to be ineffective. The injured player who suffered at the hands of an allegedly negligent act by his doctor could sue, and if this occured on a visit abroad, the injured party has the opportunity to pursue an action in the local jurisdiction. This is disadvantageous from the doctor's stand-point as in USA and Canada the levels of compensation awarded tend to be higher. It is important therefore to have insurance cover for professional liability. It is possible that your protection organisation may provide this cover even though the UK medical defence organisations do not write business in North America. Any cover would be by virtue of your UK membership but would be only likely to cover you for members of your own team or touring party. It is essential however that you check with them first, preferably in writing. As an alternative, or if you cannot get cover from your own indemnifiers, it would be reasonable to ask the World Rugby Union or whichever governing body is responsible for the sport in question to underwrite your insurance. Make no mistake however that insurance is essential.

MOLLOY: The University Medical Hospital are covered by insurance. I presumed until now that this covered me anywhere I went. The problem with touring overseas is one that we have all come across. We luckily have colleagues on site that look after us. In other words, if there is a serious injury on the field, one has a colleague from that country to protect us in more ways than one. Is this the only way that we are protected then?

PAYNE: Certainly if you are handing over the clinical management of a patient to someone else then you are no longer liable—as long as the transfer has been a clinically reasonable thing to do in the circumstances, and was a reasonable referral to the right speciality, but I am sure that would always be the case. You would be looking always at an orthopaedic surgeon I would imagine.

MOLLOY: The only other situation where there is a risk on tour is of course off the field at night and so on. What happens in that situation?

PAYNE: I suppose that would be a 'Good Samaritan' type of situation. Again, if you are providing a professional service, even as a 'Good Samaritan' you may be legally liable. There is no exemption from liability if you provide assistance—even if it is unexpected and uninvited—and you provide it in a negligent manner. There has never, to my knowledge, been a case in the UK, but I believe there have been cases in the USA. It is an extremely unlikely scenario but you cannot exclude the possibility.

18: Liability and Rugby in the USA

STEVE GRAY

IN THE field of recreation in the USA, many recreation programmes no longer exist. Some swimming programmes in California, for instance, are not offered because of the legal implications. In rugby, we are at the forefront of major changes. The first ever lawsuit in which the captain and president of a tournament organising committee, as well as the player involved, have been sued. The outcome of the court's decision could have a major effect on the game in the USA. In the past, some schools have been sued and in the state of Illinois, high school rugby is no longer permitted because of the effects of a previous law suit.

Most of the rugby clubs in the USA play on municipal grounds. If municipalities find there are going to be lawsuits, they will probably not let the teams play. Much of the way rugby is conducted in the USA is unsafe. If lawyers knew about this situation, many would immediately adjourn to the nearest rugby match and seize the opportunity to make a great amount of money! The rugby community in the USA is on the whole, naive in the area of legal liability. Clubs need to develop a comprehensive risk management programme [1]. For instance, we do not have regular rugby pitches, necessitating games being played in areas with baseball back-stops and cement obstacles on edges of the pitch. The appointment of a club officer in charge of risk management would allow him to look for possible risks, making sure these risks are systematically checked. Additionally, medical clinicians should be actively involved in risk management programmes. The first aspect of a systematic programme is to identify the risk [2].

In a typical USA programme one could potentially follow the following plan:

1 Inspect the facilities and the field. Facilities and field are typically not set up to play rugby. For example, there may be a track encircling the field. Someone thrown onto the concrete edge of the track could provide a lawyer with a lucrative pay day. A check-list might include hazards such as sprinkler heads and field conditions. One person should check the field before every practice and game to see if it is safe.

2 Check equipment. In the USA scrum machines are often archaic and dangerous and should be checked to make sure they are safe.

3 Evaluate participants' abilities and skills. One of the key problems in the USA is matching of participants. One must match participants whenever

activity involves physical collision and not merely incidental contact. Participant pairing must not ignore age, maturity, weight, height, skill and experience [3]. In the USA, a new player may be 14 years old and have never seen the game of rugby. Ten minutes later, he may be scrummaging in the front row in a practice session, or taking part in a tackling drill with no prior instruction. Americans often put their heads in front when they tackle. These practices put the club at severe risk should injury occur. Courts have also found that if a person who is large and experienced is pitted against someone who is smaller and inexperienced, one may be liable [3].

Additionally, most school programmes require physical examinations and clubs should do the same for players at the beginning of the season. Additionally, if a player is injured and not fully recovered before resuming playing in the USA, the coach or doctor could be vulnerable if a subsequent injury results. In particular, concussion followed by early resumption is especially dangerous, and coach and/or doctor could be liable in this situation.

4 Warning of inherent danger in the activity. In the USA, waivers are a common practice, although they are often meaningless in law. Sometimes an injured player does not realize he can sue despite signing the waiver and, therefore, a lawsuit can be avoided. It is important to give people verbal warning when they are about to do things that are dangerous. One needs to mention that scrummaging can be dangerous and that the right techniques must be mastered.

5 Instructing in proper techniques. New players should go through proper training. For the scrum, there should be a certified front row course. In the USA, numerous players are thrown into games with virtually no experience in the front row. It may be better to stop the game if no experienced front row players are availale. If this option is not feasible, the scrums should be conceded with no pushing allowed. If one introduces players not used to playing in a particular position and injury ensues, one may be held liable in the US courts. Suits could be filed against the referee, as well as against the coaches and the club administrators.

6 Close control of activities of play. If a referee sees the scrum collapsing time after time, or if someone is continually high-tackling, control measures need to be taken (i.e. removal from the game and/or club). Such a regular pattern of play may lead a club into disrepute. This could become an issue in the courts.

7 First aid and access to medical treatments. At every match someone who is trained in advanced first aid should be available. In the USA, the majority of states have enacted Good Samaritan statutes to encourage physicians to give prompt treatment for accident victims by excusing physicians from

civil liability in rendering emergency care [4]. The advice of local attorneys should be sought to ensure that these situations are in effect in your area. It is useful to have a manual setting out all emergency procedures. The doctor should be involved in this process.

References

1 Gray SW. Risk management in parks and recreation: need for computerized information management system. *Proc 9th Inter-Mountain Leisure Symp* 1989; 21.
2 Kraus RG, Curtis JE. *Creative Management in Recreation, Parks, and Leisure Services.* St Louis: Times Mirror/CV Mosby, 1986: 335.
3 Kaiser RA. *Liability and Law in Recreation, Parks, and Sports.* Englewood Cliffs, New Jersey: Prentice-Hall, 1986: 174.
4 Kaiser RA. *Liability and Law in Recreation Parks, and Sports.* Englewood Cliffs, New Jersey: Prentice-Hall, 1986, 182.

19: The Risks of Infection in Rugby

J.C.M.SHARP

INFECTION in sport has taken a high profile in recent years, largely due to the increasing awareness and concern about HIV infection. The Scottish Sports Council, in an attempt to put this in perspective, sponsored a booklet which covers a wide range of infections which may cause problems amongst sporting participants.

Infections may be acquired in sport in different ways. Firstly, by person-to-person spread via direct personal contact or air-borne droplets, or by blood-borne spread such as may occur with HIV and hepatitis B. Secondly, a player may become infected by contact with another infected player or contaminated changing room environment or playing-field, by insect bites or consuming contaminated food or water. Infection may be thus acquired either during sporting activity, within the changing room, during travel (particularly overseas), or as a consequence of various leisure time activities peripheral to sport.

In sporting activity, infections may be acquired by person-to-person spread or from a contaminated playing area. The contact sports, water sports and other field sports pose most risks. Infections which characterise these modes of spread are scrumpox, tetanus and other wound infections

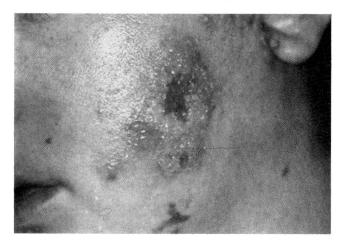

Fig. 19.1 An illustration of scrumpox occurring in a schoolboy rugby player.

and the possibility of HIV and other viral infections. Scrumpox may be caused by a range of aetiological agents which may be viral, bacterial or fungal (Fig. 19.1). These are spread by physical and abrasive contact, which is a feature of combat sports such as rugby and wrestling (Fig. 19.2). Firstly, there is the herpes form of scrumpox caused by the herpes simplex type 1 virus, not to be confused with the type 2 virus which is the cause of genital herpes. This highly infectious condition spreads very rapidly from person to person. Secondly, the impetiginous (bacterial) form of scrumpox

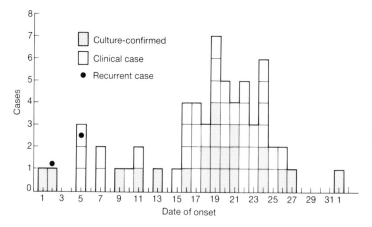

Fig. 19.2. Herpes gladiatorum cases at a high school wrestling camp by date of onset (Goodman *et al. MMWR*, 1990).

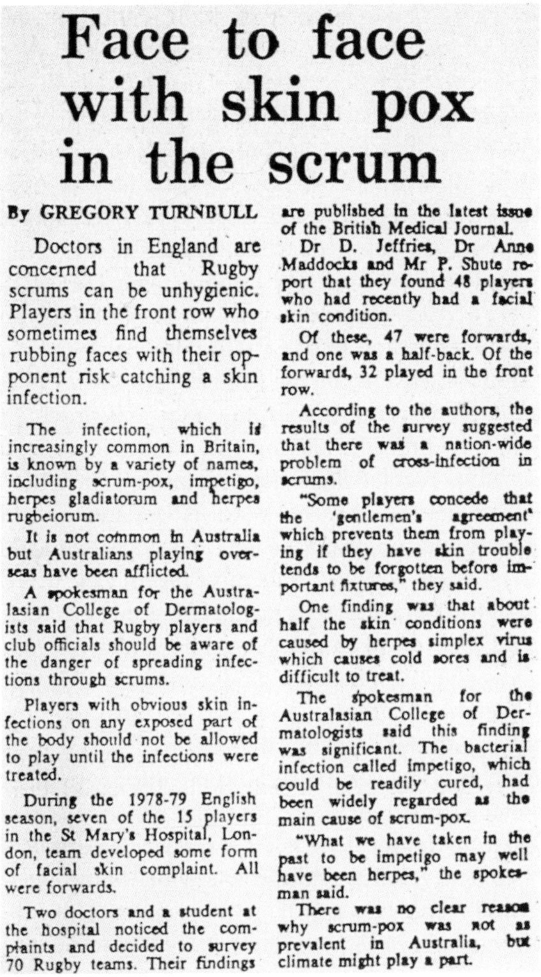

Face to face with skin pox in the scrum

By GREGORY TURNBULL

Doctors in England are concerned that Rugby scrums can be unhygienic. Players in the front row who sometimes find themselves rubbing faces with their opponent risk catching a skin infection.

The infection, which is increasingly common in Britain, is known by a variety of names, including scrum-pox, impetigo, herpes gladiatorum and herpes rugbeiorum.

It is not common in Australia but Australians playing overseas have been afflicted.

A spokesman for the Australasian College of Dermatologists said that Rugby players and club officials should be aware of the danger of spreading infections through scrums.

Players with obvious skin infections on any exposed part of the body should not be allowed to play until the infections were treated.

During the 1978-79 English season, seven of the 15 players in the St Mary's Hospital, London, team developed some form of facial skin complaint. All were forwards.

Two doctors and a student at the hospital noticed the complaints and decided to survey 70 Rugby teams. Their findings are published in the latest issue of the British Medical Journal.

Dr D. Jeffries, Dr Anne Maddocks and Mr P. Shute report that they found 48 players who had recently had a facial skin condition.

Of these, 47 were forwards, and one was a half-back. Of the forwards, 32 played in the front row.

According to the authors, the results of the survey suggested that there was a nation-wide problem of cross-infection in scrums.

"Some players concede that the 'gentlemen's agreement' which prevents them from playing if they have skin trouble tends to be forgotten before important fixtures," they said.

One finding was that about half the skin conditions were caused by herpes simplex virus which causes cold sores and is difficult to treat.

The spokesman for the Australasian College of Dermatologists said this finding was significant. The bacterial infection called impetigo, which could be readily cured, had been widely regarded as the main cause of scrum-pox.

"What we have taken in the past to be impetigo may well have been herpes," the spokesman said.

There was no clear reason why scrum-pox was not as prevalent in Australia, but climate might play a part.

Fig. 19.3. Article in the *Sydney Morning Herald* 8 January 1980.

which is caused by *Staphylococcus* or *Streptococcus pyogenes*, is still prevalent although less common than the herpes form. Erysipelas, also caused by *Streptococcus pyogenes*, is the least common form, but is clinically the most serious.

In the early 1970s several players in the 'All Blacks' touring team acquired a form of scrumpox in the south of England which spread thereafter to Irish front-row forwards. Other episodes have occurred throughout the years. An interesting comment in the *Sydney Herald* (Fig.

19.3) implied that the herpes form of scrumpox is not common in Australia, although Australians playing overseas had become infected. A rare complication of scrumpox is described as 'scrum kidney'. In December 1986 an outbreak of scrumpox affected players in the St Thomas' Hospital rugby team [1]. Following a match against an opposition where several players were found to be infected with an impetigenous form of scrumpox, five of the St Thomas' team were infected. One week later, further players in another team were also affected, while two girlfriends of the St Thomas players were also found to be infected 1 month later. This was a particularly virulent form of *Streptococcus pyogenes*; one of the girlfriends acquired acute streptococcal salpingitis and one of the original rugby players developed acute glomerulonephritis, hence the term 'scrum kidney'.

The most commonly occurring wound infections are due to organisms which are often present in the playing environment, particularly if poorly maintained. Of all sport-related infections, tetanus is the most serious and is potentially life threatening. In recent years in Scotland there have been two rugby players and one soccer player who developed clinical tetanus after cuts, only one of whom survived. The most recent case was a young man playing in a match during which he acquired a deep laceration into a finger caused by a stud. He was taken to the local hospital where the wound was cleansed. He was given Triplopen, a long-lasting penicillin, to counter the possibility of bacterial contamination. His tetanus immunisation history was technically up to date, having had his last booster exactly 10 years prior to this incident. (The current recommendations are that booster doses should be given at intervals of between 10 and 20 years.) One week after he was discharged from the accident and emergency department he developed early signs of clinical tetanus and the following day was admitted to the intensive care unit where he was put on intravenous relaxants. He survived and was discharged a month later; but it begs the question—is a 10-year interval sufficient for booster doses for rugby players and other contact sports? These circumstances suggest that perhaps it should be 5 years, but one has to remember the danger of sensitivity reactions with too frequent booster doses of tetanus toxoid.

In a recent study of 32 patients in Canada following influenza-type illnesses, 20 showed some evidence of cardiac damage [2]. The influenza A virus has been isolated from the myocardium in patients examined at postmortem, including a recent 27 year old previously healthy woman in Finland [3]. Experimental studies have been carried out showing the effect of the A virus and other viruses on the myocardium of mice. In addition to the influenza virus, some of the Coxsackie viruses can also infect and damage heart muscle. It follows that an athlete who is feverish should be resting at home in bed (watching the match on television), rather than trying to sweat it out. There are other longer term effects of viral infections on sport performance, not just the current effect of the player resuming too soon after convalescence and having a poor game, but also the longer term effects like 'post-viral (chronic) fatigue syndrome'. There is still considerable world-wide discussion about what defines this syndrome. There have been various viruses associated with this particular condition; the Coxsackie group of viruses; Epstein–Barr virus, chicken pox, measles and possibly others not yet identified.

For those travelling overseas, there is always the possibility of meeting the local 'bug', usually in conditions of poor environmental hygiene. There is no doubt that with the expansion of air travel more and more countries are being visited each year by touring sides where rare and exotic infections are more commonplace than in Europe. This is especially so of the developing countries. The majority of such infections are gastro-intestinal. Several years ago, a Scottish ladies' soccer team toured Morocco and at least four of them developed acute paratyphoid fever. Viral hepatitis type A is similarly acquired by the faecal–oral route. Respiratory infections are frequently acquired in transit—in aircraft, in terminal buildings or in hotels where the air-conditioning systems may spread infection throughout the environment.

The disease that causes most trouble and which is most likely to produce fatalities, is malaria. Despite efforts by the World Health Organisation it has increased in some countries. It is a problem which is due to developing resistance of the mosquito to DDT and other insecticides and increasing resistance of the parasite to the various drugs that are used. One particular problem in south-eastern Asia is the development of increasing resistance to both chloroquine and Fansidar. Specific up-to-date advice may change from country to country and week to week.

What can one do to protect a traveller? By and large not a great deal. While there are vaccines available against typhoid, cholera and yellow fever, most emphasis should be placed on giving advice in relation to social behaviour and what to eat and drink.

Increasing attention has been given to the hazards of HIV in recent years. The soccer World Cup of 1990 led to an increasing concern by FIFA. Various requirements were introduced such as the compulsory wearing of shinguards as a preventative measure against the potential danger of acquiring the HIV infection following injuries on the soccer field. Whether this is relevant to HIV spread is doubtful. Various other precautions have been issued such as discouraging kissing the scorer of goals and sharing a bath with team mates.

A number of different sports, not surprisingly, have reacted to the potential hazards of AIDS. In the 1989 London Marathon all persons attending to the runners were required to wear gloves. This should not have been necessary, provided that normal basic hygiene precautions were taken. By June 1990 over 266000 cases were report by 156 countries through WHO in Geneva. These figures exclude countries within the African zone who were not reporting. Bermuda has been in the top three of the highest infection rate ranking in the world; the USA is eighth, the UK 37th, with Canada and France somewhere in between. It is estimated that by the mid-1990s, 700000 cases of AIDS will have been reported world-wide.

The virus has been grown from semen, cervical secretions, lymphocytes, cell-free plasma, cerebrospinal fluid, tears, saliva, urine and breast milk. The concentration within these fluids varies widely, with semen, blood and possibly cervical secretions being particularly infectious. Unlike the hepatitis B virus, of which the routes of transmission are virtually identical, the HIV virus is not robust and does not survive for long outside the human body, although it will survive up to 3 days dried in human plasma kept at room temperature. It does not withstand exposure to heat and can be killed off by ordinary household bleach. From enquiries made world-wide within households where at least one person is known to be HIV positive, the sexual and intravenous routes apart, transfer of infection has been recorded infrequently. However, because both identified and unidentified so-called 'healthy carriers' are present on a world-wide basis in the general population, it is advisable for anyone attending an injured person to apply good hygienic practices. The unwitting transfer of the HIV or hepatitis B virus will be minimised if basic precautions are followed, particularly if there is a spillage of blood. It is known that HIV virus has been transmitted on occasion to health care workers as a consequence of needle-stick injuries, in particular from North America. World-wide, 19 such incidents have been reported.

Despite reassurances that HIV infection could not be spread by sport, a report from Italy published in the *Lancet* [4], drew attention to infection having been acquired following an injury in a football match when the head of a 25-year-old player collided with the head of another player, a known drug abuser who was HIV positive. There was severe bleeding from the eyebrows of both players, and 2 months after the incident the hitherto uninfected play was found to be HIV positive. He apparently had no known risk factors such as drug abuse or homosexual contact—he had not been in Africa or the Caribbean, was reported to have been having a stable relationship with a woman who was HIV negative for the previous 4 years, and had had no sex with other women; 1 year before he had been screened for potential military service purposes and was known then to be negative. The case was compatible with acquisition of infection by traumatic contact on the sports field with a sero-positive player. Another report in the *New England Journal of Medicine* [5], described a young French rugby player who had seroconverted and acquired early AIDS complex. As a consequence of acute tendonitis following intensive training, he had undergone a 6-week course of acupuncture. Three months later he acquired his initial illness following which the HIV positivity was found, with infection appearing to have been acquired from acupuncture.

Of all infections, HIV has the potential of being transmitted to a greater or lesser extent within all four sporting scenarios, namely, in descending order; (a) during the sporting activities; (b) in the changing room environment; (c) during travel; or (d) during leisure time activities. In consequence various sporting bodies have brought out pamphlets and advice regarding the need to improve hygiene generally within sport, but with a special reference to HIV and AIDS. In addition there are 'HIV travel kits' which can be purchased in the UK comprising needles, syringes, i.v.-giving sets and plasma expanders.

With the increasing awareness of HIV infection in relation to sport, the WHO held a meeting of experts in January 1989. The International Rugby Football Board and representatives from the International Federation of Sports Medicine and of wrestling were represented, although neither soccer nor boxing was represented. At the end of this 2-day meeting, a consensus was issued stating that on existing evidence, the spread of HIV infection appears to be unlikely as a result of normal social activities or through participation in sport. The main emphasis was on the need to improve hygiene generally—environmental as well as personal hygiene and in relation to the stopping of blood and the covering of wounds. The report did not specifically say that the communal bucket and sponge should be banned, but concern was expressed about spillage of blood and the risk of infection thus being transmitted from player to player. WHO also recommended the need to ensure that any personal cuts and scratches are covered by a waterproof dressing. In the presence of blood or abrasions, disposable gloves should be available. It was also stressed that there was no justification for pre-competitive screening or testing of athletes. However, it was suggested that any person who thought he was HIV positive should seek advice from the team doctor prior to participating, not only in relation to hazards to others, but also in relation to his own health.

Finally the need to promote education about HIV and hepatitis B within sporting organisations, was also emphasised.

References

1 Ludlam H, Cookson B. Scrum kidney: epidemic pyoderma caused by a nephritogenic *Streptococcus pyogenes* in a rugby team. *Lancet* 1986; **2**: 331.
2 Montague TJ, Marrie TJ, Bewick BJ *et al*. Cardiac effects of common viral illnesses. *Chest* 1988; **94**: 919.
3 Engblom E, Ekfors TO, Meurman DH, Toivanen A, Nikoskelainen J. Fatal influenza A myocarditis with isolation of virus from the myocardium. *Acta Med Scand* 1983; **213**: 75.
4 Torre D, Sampietro C, Ferraro G, Zeroli C, Speranza F. Transmission of HIV-1 infection via sports injury. *Lancet* 1990; **1**: 1105.
5 Vittecoq D, Mettetal JF, Rouzioux C, Bach JF, Bouchon JP. Acute HIV infection after acupuncture treatments. *N Engl J Med* 1989; **320**: 250.

Discussion

QUESTIONER: Should we be worrying about mouth-to-mouth resuscitation and the spread of AIDS through saliva? If it can be spread through body fluids why don't we worry so much about the saliva aspect—and why do dentists seem to worry about it so much?

SHARP: In this case of a dentist in California having acquired HIV through working with an infected patient it does raise that question.

CHASE: The dentist gave it to the patient!

SHARP: Saliva does carry the virus, but it appears only in very small numbers. It has been realised for some time that a fairly substantial amount of the virus is necessary to be introduced into the blood stream in mouth-to-mouth resuscitation, but we cannot say that it did not happen. By and large this should not be a major risk problem. This brings us back to the need for basic hygiene—putting something between your mouth and his mouth—a piece of gauze for example.

CHASE: I recently took a CPR [cardiopulmonary resuscitation] course from an outside concern which has gone into the business of teaching CPR. There is a big push in the new courses to say that anybody who even wants to think about doing CPR is advised to carry a one-way breathing mask which has a valve in it. They would not be criticised or expected to do CPR on an unknown victim without having one. You can see that the whole attitude is beginning to change.

MOLLOY: There is one exception—the one where the patient is bleeding in the mouth. There has been a case where a nurse was the first person at the scene of an accident and she had to give mouth-to-mouth resuscitation and she acquired the HIV virus. So rugby could be potentially dangerous.

I would also like to ask about scrumpox—once you get it, it is a latent virus and it stays there indefinitely. What is your instruction there because we tend not to let people play again until we are happy that they don't have it and there are no obvious lesions. Is there anything more specific that we can do? Is it possible therefore to let a player play who has a lesion which has appeared that day if you can cover the whole lesion?

SHARP: At that stage it is impossible to know whether it is a virus or not. It is necessary to cover the lesion as well as possible—I do not think it is very strong grounds to say that the player cannot play. Put on Betadine or something similar and cover it securely as best you can.

QUESTIONER: A point about dentists taking protection against AIDS; I understand from the British Medical Association that the recommendation to wear masks and glasses is because when they put the dental drill in the mouth, the saliva is put into an aerosol mist which can be absorbed into the mucosa.

CHASE: Two points I'd like to make—first of all the Institute of American Academy Orthopaedics is very concerned about AIDS and orthopaedic surgeons because of the bone dust and all the other things that are in the air. There was a paper given there which showed that the aerosol from the surgery floor (the second floor) was found on the sixth floor of the hospital building. So there is no question that it gets outside the theatre of surgery. The other thing is that the AIDS virus is not nearly as brittle as people originally thought it was. It does live in other situations where we didn't think it was before. Finally, did anybody know that the reported Italian player was HIV positive before he went onto the field? Did the player know?

SHARP: They were playing a team, for some reason, who were known drug-abusers.

20: Dope Testing in the Rugby World Cup

J.E.DAVIES

DO DRUGS WORK? Does placebo work? Does suggestion work? Yes, all three of them. Voltaire once said that doctors pour drugs, of which they know little, to cure diseases, of which they know less, into human beings, of whom they know nothing. There are huge ethical issues here. Some people talk very openly about legalising and allowing drugs to be used in sport. Just as violence is a form of cheating, drug abuse is certainly cheating. We have to eliminate the cheats and as far as rugby is concerned the World Cup directors have agreed that there will be randomised dope testing. The author of this chapter will be the controller and he has to organise the sampling world-wide.

Most athletes in training are no strangers to musculoskeletal inflammation, and a short course of aspirin if often of use in helping symptoms settle and expediting a return to full-time training. Commonly used agents are piroxicam, naproxen and other non-steroidal anti-inflammatories (NSAIDs). For musculoskeletal inflammatory conditions which have not responded to an adequate trial of conservative therapy, a local steroid injection may prove effective. However, since local anaesthetics are one of the classes of drugs subjected to certain restrictions, if an athlete is to have a local anaesthetic before or during a competition, some sports require a written submission of the diagnosis, the dose and the route of administration. The practice of prescribing parenteral corticosteroids to promote recovery from overtraining is not recommended. Therefore, it is a question of balance; the use of drugs for non-therapeutic purposes is both widespread and ancient [1]. Man has cultivated vines, poppies, tobacco plants and a host of other things over thousands of years, and has been seeking naturally occurring substances to improve psychomotor performance for centuries. American Indians have used cocaine to decrease hunger and improve stamina on long marches. It is thought that both third century Greek and fierce Nordic athletes ingested psychotropic mushrooms for competition. The mythology of Popeye and spinach extends back over many centuries. For the French doctors there has been the *vin moriani*, the wine of the athletes. As long ago as 1869 cyclists were using speed balls of heroin and cocaine. In 1945-50 amphetamines were 'in vogue' and were being used by racing cyclists. In the 1960s, steroids were introduced, during the 1970s testosterone and more recently growth hormone and human gonadotrophin.

Following the amphetamine-related deaths of several cyclists in the late 1960s, the International Olympic Committee set up a medical commission charged with eradicating drug abuse in Olympic sports. Testing was first introduced in the Grenoble Games in the winter of 1968, then more comprehensively in the Mexico Games the following summer.

The first Olympics during which testing for steroids took place was in Montreal in 1976. This was after the development of the reliable radio-immunoassay technique at St Thomas' Hospital in London.

Various devices have been used by athletes and their aids to enable continued drug use without the risk of disqualification. It has become a war. The term 'chemical athlete' has been introduced in recent years. Athletes can use steroids with a rapid excretion, and, as the competition approached, flush out the drug and/or use masking substances to make analysis more difficult. Athletes may also perform, or have performed for them, their own assay prior to departing for a competition and then withdraw if found to be still excreting. Other techniques rumoured to have been used include a submission of 'clean' samples from bottles left behind the cistern, from a bag in the axilla, by a fine tubing tape all the way down the body to the urethral meatus, or the allegedly stimulating but risky technique of urinary infusion in which a close friend passes urine into the catheterised bladder.

Currently, doping is defined as the administration of, or the use by, a competing athlete of any substance foreign to the body or of any physiological substance taken in abnormal quantity, or taken by an abnormal route of entry into the body with the sole intention of increasing, in an artificial manner, his or her performance in competition.

There are six different pharmacological classes of agents. There are the doping classes; stimulants, narcotics, anabolic steroids, beta-blockers, diuretics, peptide hormones and their analogues. There are three practices, and four classes of drugs subject to certain restriction; alcohol, marijuana, local anaesthetics and corticosteroids.

Stimulants, which include sympathomimetic amines and central nervous system (CNS) stimulants, have proved popular with competitors with both endurance-based sports, for example cycling, and sports requiring explosive power and aggression—field events and weightlifting.

Anecdotally, amphetamines have been used in rugby and their use may be especially prevalent in one country.

The narcotic analgesics are banned by sports governing bodies to prevent athletes competing with the pain of injury masking a situation which might lead to worse damage. They are not heavily abused by the injury-free. The use of anabolic steroids to improve performance in sport has been known for about 30 years, but have gained both momentum and notoriety during the last decade [2]. Testosterone is the basic steroid molecule on which these compounds are based. It is secreted by the interstitial cells of the testis in man, and stimulates development of the accessory sexual organs. The exogenous effect is used in pre-pubertal testicular underdevelopment and androgen is responsible for the male emotional make-up. The anabolic effect promotes nitrogen retention and increased synthesis and deposition of protein in tissues such as skeletal muscle. Modification of the side chains of the steroid molecule produces compounds such as Dianabol. These possess both enhanced anabolic potency and oral reliability. In 1889 the French physiologist Brown Sequard, believing old age and its associated dwindling of sexual powers to be reversed by agents contained in the testis, injected himself with crushed guinea pig testis. He reported to the 'Société Biologie' in Paris that these injections had proved effective but these personal observations were greeted with some hostility and scepticism. However, such was the susceptibility of the public to this suggestion that his report laid open the way to the celebrated transplantation of monkey testis slices which swept America and Europe during the 1920s and 1930s.

Probably the first use of anabolic steroids by athletes was in the 1950s when weightlifters sought to increase strength and bulk by the use of injectible synthetic testosterone. In the 1956 Olympics in Melbourne, many athletes were using Dianabol, an oral steroid with a high anabolic androgenic ratio. At this time, steroids had not yet been included on the list of banned substances by the International Olympic Committee. In 1987 the National Collegiate Athletic Association tested 720 footballers at the end of the season and suspended 21 who were marked positive. In 1988, the former British sprinter, David Jenkins, was found guilty of charges of steroid trafficking in the USA and the scale of the problem became much more apparent. In the same year at the Seoul Olympics in Korea a battle between the athletes and the biochemist was brought to the newspaper headlines of the world by the stripping of Ben Johnson.

When it comes to estimating the scale of the problem the matter becomes more complex. In former surveys of athletes, particularly those in sports requiring either great bulk and strength or explosive power, it is suggested that as many as 90% of those in serious training have used steroids at one time or another. Formal statistics are less easy to achieve; a survey of amateur body builders in a Scottish gymnasium was performed by McCulloch in 1987. Twenty per cent admitted to the use of drugs for enhancing their performance and most of these were anabolic steroids. All the users had taken combinations of drugs and in no case had there been any medical supervision.

The same problem of gathering reliable statistics for what is a widely practised but illegal activity, has also meant that any form of control of the use of steroids has been impossible. While some team physicians in the USA have said that they think steroid use is declining one experienced observer has recently stated that every professional football player takes them, with some position-related exceptions.

An excerpt from one of the weight body building journals in Britain advertises what is claimed to be a true steroid replacement. In fact steroids are widely available in gymnasiums and body building apparatus facilities in Britain.

Do anabolic steroids work? The evidence that they can in fact increase muscle mass and power is inconclusive. Lamb in 1984 revealed 19 studies in which some form of controlled trial was available. These studies showed that weight gains averaging 2.2 kg over a period of 3–12 weeks were obtained by athletes taking methandrostanolol. While some of this gain may be due to fluid retention, there was probably also a substantial increase in lean body mass. In addition, approximately half of these control investigations showed that there was a progressive improvement in muscular strength when steroids were taken along with highly intensive weight training. Athletes taking steroids typically achieve gains over those taking placebo, which average 8 g for single repetition maximum lifts in the bench press and 11 kg in the squat.

An important physiological observation must be made in relation to these studies. Those athletes who gain a major beneficial effect from the use of anabolic steroids are invariably those already engaged in the most rigorous levels of physical training. The reason for this is that the anabolic effects of exogenous steroids are intrinsically very short-lived. Thus, little or no benefit may be gained by a subject in a neutral state of metabolism. However, intensively training athletes induce in themselves a persistent catabolic state mediated by high levels of corticosteroid, resulting from increased adrenocorticotrophic hormone (ACTH) stimulation.

Finally, it must be admitted that not all the beneficial effects of anabolic steroids in training athletes are critically dependent on physiological changes. One of the principal effects reported by those using these drugs is increased physical tolerance to training and more rapid recovery from heavy training sessions. This may indeed by a physical effect, but they also have a strong psychological component. Moreover, the increased aggress-iveness which is undoubtedly one of the effects of steroids may itself make a major contribution to the athlete's performance. A search for evidence from control trials for or against the physical effects of steroids is doomed to failure. Most clinical trials in medicine are aimed at demonstrating differences between groups of at least 10%. By contrast, an improvement in performance of only 1–2% may represent the margin between victory and defeat in international athletic events.

The side effects of steroids can take place in the cardiovascular system; they can cause fluid retention which may in part account for the early weight gain during their use. Significant increases in blood pressure occur, along with left ventricular hypertrophy and changes in lipoproteins have been observed during several studies in training athletes. Many steroids increase the level of clotting factors—particularly factors V, X and prothrombin. In the male reproductive system testosterone and its analogues cause suppression of follicular-stimulating hormone and luteinising hormone. This results in testicular atrophy, oligo- and azospermia. Gynaecomastia is a frequent finding; one paper reported 38 surgical procedures for this condition in body builders in the USA. In the female reproductive system, side effects of steroids include uterine atrophy and menstrual irregularity which are common, making pregnancy unlikely. However, if steroids are taken during pregnancy, pseudo-hermaphrodism or fetal death are both hazards. Amongst secondary sexual changes in women, acne, deepening of the voice, facial hair and baldness, shrinking of the breasts and clitoral hypertrophy contribute to the features. Major stimulation of the sebaceous glands occur in either sex. Effects in children include premature fusion and permanent stunting of growth. In adolescence, extreme virilisation may occur along with gynaecomastia. The psychological effects include mood swings and unpredictable, aggressive behaviour. There have been reports of criminal activities resulting from psychological disturbances. Abnormal results of liver function tests whilst taking steroids are common, with increased transaminases and alkaline phosphatase. In severe cases a cholestatic hepatitis may occur. These changes are not generally reversible on withdrawal of steroids and have to be distinguished from the elevation of transaminases which may occur with intense weight lifting alone. There have also been reports of hepatomas of the liver.

The steroid users, the 'chemical athletes', are clever. They are not medically qualified but they read the literature [3]. Sophisticated patterns of drug taking have evolved in order to maximise gains, keep side effects to a minimum and beat the drug tests. Steroids are usually taken in cycles of between 4 and 12 weeks to enable endogenous testosterone levels and pancreatic function tests (PFTs) to return to normal between cycles. 'Stacking' involves the taking of two drugs simultaneously. 'Short gunning' is the dubious practice of taking several preparations at once, and there are also 'plateauing' and 'staggering'. In Wales, young men ingested chicken pellets because they contain very low doses of steroids. They were given these in gymnasiums. Athletes usually do obtain these drugs from the black market, although steroids remain freely available under-the-counter in some countries.

Growth hormone became popular in the late 1970s and 1980s due to the more rapid and more permanent gains it was alleged to produce in combination with its undetectability. The Sports Council in Wales had an enormous row with a Welsh Ladies Bowls Association because the majority were taking beta-blockers. They wanted to legislate and allow for beta-blockers to be allowed. The answer was definitely no. Probenecid is used to suppress the urinary excretion of certain drugs prior to competition, i.e. as a masking agent, and prolactin may be used to increase appetite and facilitate weight gain. Thyroxine is sometimes used to assist weight loss and ACTH may assist in recovery from overtraining and inflammatory problems. Blood doping was given wide exposure by Mr Virren who attributed his 5000 and 10000 metre victories to reindeer milk.

The detection of drugs used to enhance sporting performance has become a new major industry [4]. Workers at the Olympic analytical laboratory at Los Angeles reported in 1987 that they had conducted 8000 tests for androgenic anabolic steroids over a 3-year period and found several hundred positive cases. The same authors noted that during the 1984 Los Angeles Olympic Games, almost 10000 analyses were performed during a 15-day period covering more than 200 different drugs and metabolites, with only a 2% positivity rate. It has been pointed out that the drug testing facilities used for the 1984 Olympic Games cost more to operate than the total athletic budget of many countries.

The scope and nature of drug testing athletes has received increasing attention during the last decade. The publicity surrounding the Seoul Olympics in 1988 has sharpened both public and medical attention.

There are 16 countries partaking in the rugby World Cup. The approved laboratories will be in London, Paris, Tokyo, Sydney and Montreal. A global cover for randomised dope testing will be available before men come to the rugby World Competition itself.

It is a 32-match schedule, there are 19 different venues in the five nations with about 400 players. The testing programme will be from 1st August to 20 September. In the early part of August, once the squads have been chosen, a random selection of participating unions will be nominated for drug testing and there will be two players from each union. Sampling officers will come to these countries and they will be spot-checked during squad training sessions. Urine samples will be sent to the relevant laboratories world-wide.

During the tournament assembly period all teams are to be tested, two players from each team, and then again in October. During the tournament, two players from each team will be tested after each match.

In Wales, during the season 1990–91, the Welsh Rugby Union in conjunction with the Sports Council for Wales instituted the most comprehensive drug testing programme in world rugby, involving not only international squad players at all ages, but also at club level.

To assist players to abide by the IOC list of banned substances, the Sports Council for Wales have issued a small card which has been distributed by the Welsh Rugby Union so that each player is aware of what he should and should not be taking.

The International Rugby Board have indicated that they will follow the IOC list of banned substances and penalty and sanction recommendations in the event of a positive dope test.

During the Rugby World Cup competition, a positive test will result in the player being banned from the competition with no replacement being allowed. His case will then be dealt with by his own rugby union governing body.

Discussion

ENGLISH DOCTOR: To come back to the question of drugs in sport—currently the main thrust about not taking drugs is that it's cheating. There seems to be very little mention about the fact that drugs are *dangerous* for athletes to take. The Sports Council spends £600 000 a year on drug control. £50 000 of that is spent on education, and the bulk of that education is introducing booklets saying 'thou shalt not take this'. I feel very sorry about the fact that somebody is not undertaking an educational programme to try and change the climate of opinion in sport about taking drugs. You could do it through the punitive programme which is in place at the moment but the main message coming says 'you will not take these drugs because it is cheating'. There is little mention of health risk.

BATH DOCTOR: I think that 3 to 4 weeks is the length of time after which traces of steroids may have gone for obvious reasons the authorities are reluctant to specify any length of time. The current advice out of the lab is that it is becoming easier to detect smaller and smaller quantities. Therefore it is very difficult to specify the length of time that traces of steroids stay in the body.

DAVIES: Well, as an international organisation we can actually press this point about the side effects of drugs. I am glad you brought this up because I would like to ask advice from opinions around the world. The Japanese—do you suspect that any of your players are on steroids?

KUNO: I interviewed every athlete on our team, and I am sure that none of them takes steroids.

DAVIES: Can I ask you another question then, because there are cultural differences with regard to treatments in Japan compared to those in the Western Hemisphere. Are there any chemicals which the players might take for colds or influenza which may contain a banned substance?

KUNO: We have regimens for easily available drugs. Sometimes these drugs contain ephedrine. I'd like to ask you about what happens when a player takes these kinds of drugs—how do you penalise a player who takes such a popular drug?

DAVIES: The rugby authorities have not yet decided on any penalty in the event of a positive drug test. One recommendation that will have to come out of this conference for the International Rugby Board is that they must act now. If somebody is found positive in a drug test in the rugby World Cup with 150 million other people watching then the roof will go up.

WELSH QUESTIONER: During one summer there was an athlete who had been using drugs whilst shot-putting. Suddenly he decided that he wanted to play rugby in the winter—should he be banned automatically because he took drugs while he was an athlete?

DAVIES: The answer is yes. You can't let him take drugs for one sport and then let him off for another.

ENGLAND: You mentioned in your address that there was one South American country which was very concerned about the problems of drug taking amongst its players. Indeed they are very concerned about it and they were waiting to see what the IRB was going to do about pre-tournament doping. They were interested to hear that it was hoped that 6 months testing would be done prior to tournament and they are going to do this anyway because they intend to stamp this out.

A point about penalties for this—they know which province is involved and they are looking for guidance about what to do should they find the players positive. I had to say that I didn't know. They're going to wait to see what the Rugby Football Union or other unions decide. There are two opportunities here, first of all, we have to provide very strong recommendations. Secondly, individual unions will not move until they see what others are going to do because there may be many implications.

DAVIES: Individuals are not going to move until they get the directive from the International Rugby Board. There has been correspondence between them and us for the last 5 months—in fact we have been pleading with them but they have just been ignoring us.

GRAYSON: Every other international organisation, whether it is the IOC, the IAAF, FIFA, etc., have got their sanctions which are essential just as any road traffic law is valueless unless you have the penalties as a result of the convictions.

DAVIES: In Wales we have started a very random drug testing programme. Do we go along with the International Olympic Committee guide-lines for 2 years and then life, or do we follow the International Sports Federation Guide-lines which are slightly different for different subjects, or do we introduce our own?

GRAYSON: Provided it is fair and reasonable and not outrageously disproportionate to the offence, any governing body which is itself autonomous is justified in introducing its own sanction level.

WELSH QUESTIONER: Do we introduce our own list of drugs then or do we go along with the IOC?

BATH DOCTOR: Can I suggest that the IOC list (although it is the best list that there is), the actual facts about whether or not drugs can enhance performance are not really sufficiently well established at the moment. I think there is a danger if you try and produce your own list in a hurry then you could end up with more problems. I would suggest that we utilise the IOC list which everybody is familiar with. Although there are drawbacks to this, and it does penalize medical treatment in some ways, nevertheless it is a tried, improved list and it is probably better to do it through a body like that.

DAVIES: I would accept that, and if I could put that to you now that one of the recommendations would be for you to look at this. Consider using the IOC recommendations—both on the list of drugs and also on penalties.

HUGO: There is some discrepancy because I'm not quite sure if all the bodies use exactly the same penalty code. I think the athletic people have come up with some decisions, and I think they're the first body who would allow (and the gentlemen who were involved with this can verify it) that you now can say if there is a particular athlete which you want to be tested—he would then be tested by the national body. I think by following the athletic field we do not have to re-invent the wheel. If we look at their penalties for something like steroids there is a penalty for about 2 years and for other stimulants I think a year.

DAVIES: The easiest thing would be to follow these guide-lines.

MOLLOY: The Rugby World Cup is separate from the International Board. They are running this competition.

DAVIES: But they are still coming under the rules and regulations of the

International Rugby Board. The Rugby World Cup Board have made recommendations in the event of positive drug testing but are only going so far as saying that if a man is found positive that he would be eliminated from the Rugby World Cup competition and any subsequent Rugby World Cup competition.

GIBSON: Is there any evidence that there is a doping problem in the world of rugby? Is it possible that the Board could encourage the problem by heightening awareness?

ENGLISH DOCTOR: Can I just comment on this. The world of athletics is an outstanding example of a governing body closing its eyes to a problem until it got so out of control that there was no other way of dealing with it than by the strict regulations that they have produced. Although there may not be a problem in rugby at the moment I think it is as well to anticipate that there may be and set some machinery in place.

DAVIES: I think that there is another political issue here as well, because in most of the countries in the world the grants given to the grounds to play rugby are supplied by the sports councils. During the Rugby World Cup the Sports Councils of England and Wales said that if the rules of the International Board were not followed then they would receive no grants. It is basically blackmail, but it has to be considered.

BURRY: Can I comment that in Sydney recently one of the rugby league clubs was concerned with the end performance of their team. They decided to drug test and found that 14 men were tested positive. Out of a squad of about 20 it seemed that most of them were smoking pot, but two of them testing positive for cocaine as well. I do not think they had tested them for anabolic steroids.

They attempted to take action on this issue and the one player who had a large amount of cocaine in his system was thrown out of the club. The boy was outraged and spoke to the press about what a dreadful thing this was and his legal adviser subsequently took action against the governing body and the club. His objection to being thrown out of the club was sustained by the court. He was finally given a very large sum of money because he had a contract with the club and he then joined another club.

ENGLAND: Surely in any contract with a sporting individual he is required to present himself as being fit to play for the club if he is playing in a professional sporting activity?

BURRY: I do not think they were able to show that his performance had necessarily been impaired by drug taking.

GRAYSON: In view of this, any governing body should include in the rules the incidence of a positive dope test disqualifies the player from being under the jurisdiction of the body or the club.

BURRY: As there were no rules, that club had no right to attempt to restrain him and his activities.

MOLLOY: It is very difficult to expect every rugby player around the world to be innocent of drug taking if so many people in society take drugs.

DAVIES: The fact that you have all come here from 13 countries from around the world is tremendous. The game is rapidly developing and now it is one of the highest profile team games in the world. This is why things have to be right for this next Rugby World Cup. I see the fact that recommendations coming here, which obviously have to be channelled the correct way, not only the International Rugby Board but also to your own unions, is the right and proper way to do it. I think to carry more weight would be the setting up of an association of rugby doctors. There are one or two ideas which have been floating around and I know that John Chase and Mick Molloy have put their heads together about possibly setting up an international college of rugby medicine. All the societies, such as the Kento Medical Society in Japan, the Argentinians and so on, all the societies can be linked in to this international college. John, could you elaborate on this.

CHASE: I haven't had the opportunity to develop this in any detail but we want to have an association. Whatever recommendations we make from this meeting, we would want to be viewed as a help to rugby, and not as a thorn in the side of the game by some people who are administrators or doctors. I think there is some delicacy there. If we set this up as a scientific college that studies the incidence and the mechanisms of injury then we can use various countries as 'chapters' of that organisation.

We can get to a point where we can ask for abstract papers to be presented at scientific meetings; we can ask different countries to study aspects of the game, rather than all of us studying all the aspects of the game at the same time.

We can use our resources more effectively that way and come up with better recommendations, I think. It also gives every person who is interested in rugby an opportunity to go out to some professional association. Theoretically, it would raise the standard of care among all the people dealing with rugby and so that they are not exposed to the liability that we talked about today by being aware of the standard of care expected. These are some of the earlier views.

DAVIES: Mick, do you have any further points?

MOLLOY: It was a very brief discussion and I would certainly think that is the way it should be developed. Possibly the Welsh Association of Sports Trainers could meet at the same time so that we could exchange views. Our association needs to be integrated in a scientific way, and we should have each countries' associations as part of it and we should have these meetings and discuss the problems.

DAVIES: Does anybody else have any ideas on setting up an organisation?

HUGO: I think that the correct way of doing this is that we all agree on the principles, then we set up, or nominate, the steering committee. We need to set up the name, formulate an aim and objectives, suggest membership. This can be circulated and we can get together and perhaps formulate this whole thing by the time of the World Cup.

DAVIES: Perhaps I can go one step further and make a suggestion to you as a conference, that the steering committee being approved by you here to look into the whole issue. I would suggest that the steering committee could be the four chairman of this meeting. Also I think we should have Mr Hugo in South Africa, and Mr Kono in Japan because they have an 8 or 9 year experience at the Kento Medical Society, having already set it up. I think that six of us, unless people feel it should be different, should look at this during the next day or so while we are here. Any objections? No?

A final thing if you have any further thoughts on the matter then you leave them with the six men I have already mentioned. We will look at these and circulate material to you.

I would like to thank you all again for coming and helping us to enjoy this conference. With the five nations from France, England, Wales, Scotland, and Ireland; United States; Canada; Fiji; New Zealand; Japan; Australia and Bermuda you have all been here, and it has been great meeting you all. I would also like to thank the sponsors of the meeting— without them this would not have been possible.

References

1 Anstiss T. Uses and abuses of drugs in sport, the athletes view. In: Payne SDW, ed. *Medicine, Sport and the Law.* Oxford: Blackwell Scientific Publications, 1990: 89–91.
2 Benjamin JS. The case against anabolic steroids. In: Payne SDW, ed. *Medicine, Sport and the Law.* Oxford: Blackwell Scientific Publications, 1990: 124–31.
3 Anstiss T. Uses and abuses of drugs in sport, the athlete's view. In: Payne SDW, ed. *Medicine, Sport and the Law.* Oxford: Blackwell Scientific Publications, 1990: 96.
4 Benjamin JS. The case against anabolic steroids. In: Payne SDW, ed. *Medicine, Sport and the Law.* Oxford: Blackwell Scientific Publications, 1990: 130–1.

PART 5
INTERNATIONAL TOURING

21: International Rugby Tour Experiences

BEN GILFEATHER

IN THE last decade, the numbers of international rugby tours, and also tours undertaken by clubs (senior and junior) has escalated dramatically.

I had been acting as Medical Officer for Wasps Rugby Football Club for 15 years before being nominated as Honorary Medical Officer to the Rugby Football Union, and since 1987 I have accompanied England (1987 World Cup) and British Lions (1989) to Australia.

Prior to touring, each player has to have a medical and dental health check, for insurance purposes, and also of course, to ensure that he is not carrying an injury. The first experience of this was the day before departure for the World Cup 1987. The reserve hooker had sprung a rib cartilage 2 weeks previously in the Club's Cup Final at Twickenham. He had to be put through a rigorous check to ensure he could play. Two weeks is often not long enough for these rib cartilages and I wonder about what thresholds of pain players are prepared to endure to disguise difficulty.

A similar situation confronted me with two players prior to departure on the Lions Tour of 1989. One had badly ruptured a calf muscle 3 weeks previously playing for England in Romania, and the other had severe bilateral tibial periostitis which had caused him a lot of pain. However, after being fitted with an orthosis for over-pronating feet, he was recovering after a period of rest from rugby. Both were able to complete a full days fitness assessment along with the rest of the squad, and I was able to tell the manager that as far as their injuries were concerned, they had healed, but that their fitness needed working on.

It is vitally important that the team's medical officer is fully familiar with all immunisation requirements for those countries of the world being visited, and to ensure that these are completed well before departure.

All players must keep their anti-tetanus immunisation up to date throughout their playing careers.

A great deal has been written about jet lag and how it can affect people in a variety of ways. The further the distance travelled, generally speaking, the worse the effects can be. Certainly, when travelling to Australia and New Zealand, a minimum of 7 days, and preferably 10 days, should be allowed. Players should be advised not to drink alcohol during the flight, and also to try to take a little regular exercise every hour or so, when practical.

Probably the most difficult thing to do on tour is to tell someone that they can no longer participate because of injury, and that they have to return home. This is made all the more poignant, when it happens in training even before the first game.

Days before the inaugural match of the World Cup vs. Australia, one of the forward's knee 'broke down' in training, and he damaged a meniscus. This had to be repaired on his return home. This of course adds extra pressure on the selectors, because the replacement has to be allowed time to acclimatize, and the timing of matches becomes crucial.

In Brisbane, England vs. Australia, after 5 minutes of the match, the English full-back was knocked unconscious for 4 minutes, and in the Lions match against Western Australia in Perth in 1989, the fly-half damaged his knee in what appeared a very innocuous incident. However, he had an immediate haemarthrosis, and at operation, on his return home he had damaged his meniscus and also sustained a partial tear of his anterior cruciate ligament.

Generally speaking, the medical officer will be given every co-operation and courtesy from his opposite number, when he needs to call on them for help, e.g. X-rays or a consultant opinion. The liaison officer can be most helpful in directing the medical officer and the injured player to the nearest, most suitable hospital. The medical help given by Australian doctors and the facilities of their hospitals was first-class.

Before the Lions first test against Australia we lost a winger with a strained medial collateral ligament. This in itself is normally not too difficult to manage on tour, but his case was aggravated by the fact that he had previously completely ruptured his posterior cruciate, and he had needed extra strong musculature to stabilize the joint. He wasn't able to maintain the tone and strength he required, and he felt the knee unstable.

It is well known that injury on the rugby field can be very fickle and it has no regard for time or place. As an example, during the *last* match of the Lions tour, a centre and winger simultaneously, but in different incidents and different parts of the field, sustained full anterior dislocations of their shoulders. It could so easily have been the game before the first test. Because we were all flying home together the following day, it didn't matter, but had it happened 2–3 weeks sooner, the selectors would have had the problem of deciding as to whether to bring replacements to the other end of the earth.

It must be rare for any team medical officer on tour not to have to replace at least one player.

A problem facing all tour doctors is the attitude of some players to disguise and hide underlying injury, for fear of missing out on a tour, or another cap, and then of course, the possibility that they could lose their place to the replacement.

The pressures on the players are enormous, and are ever increasing each season, and I can well understand their fears, but cannot medically condone it because as we all know, if we treat problems early, we can invariably cure the situation before anything serious occurs. This is a problem I feel that will always be with us.

Fortunately, the vast majority of injuries are classed as mild to moderate, and each touring team needs to have a very experienced physiotherapist. Not only one who is knowledgeable, but one who is dedicated to the job in hand, and this often entails treating each injured player two to three times daily and fitting treatment sessions in with airports, hotels, etc. Doctors can learn so much from working with their physiotherapists.

It is essential to try and learn, to some degree, other skills in order to help out with the work load, as the tour progresses, by taping joints, manipulating backs, necks and massage. I feel that medical officers can only of course learn a little of these skills, because they have no formal training, but there is no truer saying than 'every little helps'.

On the two tours to Australia, I had 100 medical consultations in 1987, and 150 in 1989. One-third of these cases were of a general medical nature, and fortunately were minor in all cases. Upper respiratory infections, ear infections, some diarrhoea and skin problems, were the most frequent. The most serious medical conditions *always* occur in the attending press corps, e.g. irregular heart rates, strangulated hernia, hypertensive crisis, acute asthmatic attacks.

Each tour doctor must take with him those drugs that he feels he is most likely to need, and with which he is most familiar. From a personal view point, I feel an experienced family doctor, with experience in diagnosing and managing sports injuries, is the most suitable doctor to tour. Immediately after the last game and before departure home, each player must be examined to ensure that he is free from injury and able to play rugby football. Any player sustaining injury on tour and requiring medical care is covered by the host union's insurance.

My very first overseas rugby tour was with the Wasps when we travelled to Kenya in 1973. I made the mistake of putting my medical degrees on the tour brochure, which preceded our arrival in Kenya, and I have a degree in obstetrics and gynaecology. When we arrived up-country, on disembarking from the team-coach, a message went out for the team-doctor to come and see three women who had kept their gynaecological problems for his arrival. Who was I to refuse?

Touring is a mixture of all the emotions—excitement, fun, tension, boredom (airports, hotel-rooms, etc.) but most certainly an experience not to be forgotten.

[143]

22: A Personal Account of French Touring Experiences

JEAN PENE

I HAVE been the French Rugby Team doctor for about 20 years. The first tour I made as team doctor was to Australia in 1972. Since then I have been to New Zealand, Australia, South Africa, Fiji, but also to North and South America, Japan, Russia, Poland, Romania, Spain, Italy, North Africa— often several times in each country.

I was the first doctor appointed as an official management member of a touring team. It was in 1975 on the South African tour, that I escorted a company of about 30 people, whose main quality is not speaking English fluently. That is why I have much additional work to do; to help them and especially the manager for room accommodation, shopping, and relationships with local people including local girls.

I organise the menus. I discuss this with the chef to ensure that dishes approximate to what we are used to eating and drinking in France. We usually prefer red wine than tea and rare meat to boiled meat.

The main difference between a tour and a five-nation tournament is the period we stay out of France and consequently the quantity of medical gear I have to take with me. On a 30-day tour, I take with me three big trunks containing plenty of elastoplast tapes, medicines, surgical gear for small injuries, vitamins, antibiotics, anti-inflammatories and also aspirins. We have one condom on the field and I keep many in my trunk.

The physiotherapist travelling with me brings with him all the trunks including physiotherapy equipment. All that makes us almost autonomous but everywhere I receive a warm welcome from local doctors. I am a radiologist. The only difficulties I have to solve during tours have been radiological. It is difficult to find a radiologist on Saturday nights and most of the time I have to run the X-ray equipment and to read my results.

It takes about 3 days to resolve the effects of jet lag and not, as they used to say, 1 day for 1 hour.

The problems which occur can be classified into two groups: traumatic and medical. Injury on tours is similar in location and severity to that during ordinary games in Europe. The lower limb is most often affected especially the ankle (38%), then upper limb, especially shoulder, rib and fingers (27%), then head and face (21%), and vertebral column (8.5%). I have not seen serious neck injuries on tour.

Medical problems may include influenza, tonsillitis, gastro-intestinal symptoms and once, a case of appendicitis and one instance of viral hepatitis. During each tour I have had to send back home one player injured or seriously sick. On the last tour to Australia one player died. He succumbed to respiratory inhalation.

Rugby tours in my opinion should be shorter. Players coming home from a long tour at the end of the championship have only a very short holiday time before the next championship. It is impossible for a player to maintain fitness all year without breaks. During the last World Cup injuries occurred often during training and why not during games? Mouthguards should be compulsory.

Discussion

DAVIES: I'd like to ask Dr Pene information for all of us here. I understand that all French players have a licence. Is that correct?

PENE: Yes. If they want to play they must have a licence.

DAVIES: An insurance licence?

PENE: Yes. Insurance cover, even for international games. It is private insurance for treatment.

DAVIES: And that is where you get your statistics from.

PENE: Yes. We get the statistics from the company.

O'BRIEN: Could I ask Ben Gilfeather about the comment he made about athletes travelling with hidden injuries. I've worked with the Olympics team for quite a long time and we always assess them before they go out and anybody who has a suspected problem has to have a medical examination prior to leaving. Anyone with a history of even a minor injury must have a medical and must be fully recovered before they go.

GILFEATHER: That's absolutely right but I'm dealing with people who haven't enlightened us of their history of injury. They are carrying something which is causing pain but they are still able to play with a certain amount of pain—even at the highest levels—without us knowing about it.

O'BRIEN: But do you, as a general rule, examine all of your players at one time part of the season from a biomechanical point of view?

GILFEATHER: No.

O'BRIEN: We do, and by this means discover many minor injuries earlier.

GILFEATHER: I'd defy you to pick up all degrees of problems clinically.

WALKDEN: I think that is true. We're dealing with different forms of athleticism—rugby versus 400 metre treadmill tests.

O'Brien: I'm actually talking about rugby players.

Walkden: There is always somebody who will beat the system and they'll be on that plane for the sheer exhilaration of collecting another cap.

Gilfeather: One of the difficulties as you well know, certainly before the England departure for Australia for the World Cup, was the decision that you and I had to take on one of the hookers. The thing I found very bad about that was that the decision had to be taken at the eleventh hour. We had a substitute with his passport and his suitcase and he had to go back to his car at Twickenham and drive home. I wonder about the advisability of that and whether or not a decision should have been taken at least a week beforehand.

Chase: I just wanted to underscore the point that Ben is making—we had two players sent home from the airport on our last tour and I earlier referred to the injured reserve list that we now have whenever a player comes back from a tour. If he's injured in any way he's on the list and he has to clear that list with a medical examination. One of our biggest problems has been that even though we have a system that everyone is supposed to adhere to, invariably there will be two or three players selected in the last week before the tour leaves. So they come without a history and examination.

Walkden: For so many years we've been in an advisory capacity rather than an authoritative capacity.

Sharp: Jean—home sickness from psychological factors—to what extent is this a problem for French players in an English-speaking country?

Pene: I think that's very important but they can now ring home every day.

APPENDIX

Recommendations of the Bermuda Conference

1 Referees, coaches and teachers and other non-playing designates to have certified training in first aid, including cardiopulmonary resuscitation (CPR) and the recognition of concussion.

2 That referees should be compelled to ensure that the current laws are adhered to by players at all levels of the game and most especially at the highest level and where players' safety is at risk.

3 Conference has verified the high incidence of injuries to the tackler and ball carrier, and these include the high incidence of brain and neck injuries. The safe and correct technique in tackling and falling by coaches and teachers must be re-emphasized.

4 Rugby injury surveys to be standardised as a matter of urgency according to a common protocol and nomenclature under the International Rugby Board (IRB).

5 *IB Resolution 5.7* which states that a player who has suffered definite concussion 'should not participate' in any match or training for a period of at least 3 weeks from the time of the injury, and then only subject to being cleared by a proper neurological examination. The 'should not participate' to be reworded to '*must* not participate'.

Note. A distinction must be made between head injury in general and brain damage (concussion).

6 Conference has identified the high incidence of injuries due to foul play and emphasised the responsibility and civil and criminal legal liability of rugby authorities. Foul play *must* be severely punished and the frequent offender must not be selected.

7 Civil liability incurred by doctors providing their professional services in the management of rugby injuries was identified by the Conference as a significant risk to practitioners, especially where services are provided in, or around a match situation; playing, training or touring. Ethical dilemmas within the doctor–patient relationship arising from the possibility of an ambiguous allegiance between the doctor, his patient and the club, were also considered. The IRB is called upon to clarify (and regularise) the relationship between the team and its medical attendant and to make adequate provision for professional indemnity arrangements where necessary.

Appendix

8 The IRB *forthwith* should develop, agree and advertise to all members and associate member unions, rules including penalties and sanctions relating to the use and abuse of drugs and prohibitive substances. Conference recommended that the IOC guide-lines be adhered to.

9 Conference confirmed the potential risk of the transferral of hepatitis B virus and HIV. Players must not be allowed to compete with open bleeding wounds which cannot effectively be covered by an impermeable dressing.

Note. Contagious lesions such as scrumpox are included in this recommendation.

10 Conference identified the risk of febrile illness specifically affecting the cardiovascular system. Players who are ill or febrile *must not* be allowed to compete.

Index

Index

spinal injuries
  acute anterior spine syndrome, 34–5
  evaluation, 31–42
  rehabilitation units, 36–7
  South Africa survey, 18–22
  see also neck injuries
spondarthritis, 34
spondylolysis (spinal), 34, 39
steroids, 37
  in acute soft tissue injury, 78
  steroid abuse, 126–37
stretchers, 15, 26, 35
surveys
  value of, 3–5
    discussion, 9–11
  see also epidemiology

tackling
  injuries due to, 6–8, 28
  recommendations for, 28, 34
testosterone, 128
tetanus, 117–20

viral infections, 120–1
  HIV, 117–18, 121–3
  scrumpox, 117–20, 124–5, 150

wound infections, 120